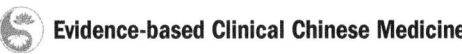 Evidence-based Clinical Chinese Medicine

Volume 29
Cervical Radiculopathy

Evidence-based Clinical Chinese Medicine

Print ISSN: 2529-7562
Online ISSN: 2529-7554

Series Co Editors-in-Chief

Charlie Changli Xue *(RMIT University, Australia)*
Chuanjian Lu *(Guangdong Provincial Hospital of Chinese Medicine, China)*

Published

Vol. 1   *Chronic Obstructive Pulmonary Disease*
          by Charlie Changli Xue and Chuanjian Lu

Vol. 2   *Psoriasis Vulgaris*
          Lead Authors: Claire Shuiqing Zhang and Jingjie Yu

Vol. 3   *Chronic Urticaria*
          Lead Authors: Meaghan Coyle and Jingjie Yu

Vol. 4   *Adult Asthma*
          Lead Authors: Johannah Shergis and Lei Wu

Vol. 5   *Allergic Rhinitis*
          Lead Authors: Claire Shuiqing Zhang and Qiulan Luo

Vol. 6   *Herpes Zoster and Post-herpetic Neuralgia*
          Lead Authors: Meaghan Coyle and Haiying Liang

Vol. 7   *Insomnia*
          Lead Authors: Johannah Shergis and Xiaojia Ni

Vol. 8   *Alzheimer's Disease*
          Lead Authors: Brian H May and Mei Feng

Vol. 9   *Vascular Dementia*
          Lead Authors: Brian H May and Mei Feng

Vol. 10   *Diabetic Kidney Disease*
          Lead Authors: Johannah Shergis and Lihong Yang

Vol. 11   *Acne Vulgaris*
          Lead Authors: Meaghan Coyle and Haiying Liang

More information on this series can also be found at https://www.worldscientific.com/series/ebccm

(Continued at end of book)

Evidence-based Clinical Chinese Medicine

Co Editors-in-Chief

Charlie Changli Xue
RMIT University, Australia

Chuanjian Lu
Guangdong Provincial Hospital of Chinese Medicine, China

Volume 29

Cervical Radiculopathy

Lead Authors

Claire Shuiqing Zhang
RMIT University, Australia

Dihui Zhang
Guangdong Provincial Hospital of Chinese Medicine, China

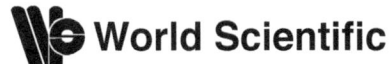

World Scientific

NEW JERSEY · LONDON · SINGAPORE · BEIJING · SHANGHAI · HONG KONG · TAIPEI · CHENNAI · TOKYO

Published by

World Scientific Publishing Co. Pte. Ltd.

5 Toh Tuck Link, Singapore 596224

USA office: 27 Warren Street, Suite 401-402, Hackensack, NJ 07601

UK office: 57 Shelton Street, Covent Garden, London WC2H 9HE

Library of Congress Cataloging-in-Publication Data
Names: Xue, Charlie Changli, author. | Lu, Chuan-jian, 1964– author.
Title: Evidence-based clinical Chinese medicine / Charlie Changli Xue, Chuanjian Lu.
Description: New Jersey : World Scientific, 2016. | Includes bibliographical references and index.
Identifiers: LCCN 2015030389| ISBN 9789814723084 (v. 1 : hardcover : alk. paper) |
    ISBN 9789814723091 (v. 1 : paperback : alk. paper) |
    ISBN 9789814723121 (v. 2 : hardcover : alk. paper) |
    ISBN 9789814723138 (v. 2 : paperback : alk. paper) |
    ISBN 9789814759045 (v. 3 : hardcover : alk. paper) |
    ISBN 9789814759052 (v. 3 : paperback : alk. paper)
Subjects: | MESH: Medicine, Chinese Traditional--methods. | Clinical Medicine--methods. |
    Evidence-Based Medicine--methods. | Psoriasis. | Pulmonary Disease, Chronic Obstructive.
Classification: LCC RC81 | NLM WB 55.C4 | DDC 616--dc23
LC record available at http://lccn.loc.gov/2015030389

Volume 29: Cervical Radiculopathy
ISBN 978-981-122-858-2 (hardcover)
ISBN 978-981-123-547-4 (paperback)
ISBN 978-981-122-859-9 (ebook for institutions)
ISBN 978-981-122-860-5 (ebook for individuals)

British Library Cataloguing-in-Publication Data
A catalogue record for this book is available from the British Library.

For any available supplementary material, please visit
https://www.worldscientific.com/worldscibooks/10.1142/12050#t=suppl

Disclaimer

The information in this monograph is based on systematic analyses of the best available evidence for Chinese medicine interventions both historical and contemporary. Every effort has been made to ensure accuracy and completeness of the data of this publication. This book is intended for clinicians, researchers and educators. The practice of evidence-based medicine consists of consideration of the best available evidence, practitioners' clinical experience and judgment, and patients' preference. Not all interventions are acceptable in all countries. It is important to note that some of the substances mentioned in this book may no longer be in use, may be toxic, or be prohibited or restricted under the provisions of the Convention on International Trade in Endangered Species of Wild Fauna and Flora (CITES). Practitioners, researchers and educators are advised to comply with the relevant regulations in their country and with the restrictions on the trade in species included in CITES appendices I, II and III. This book is not intended as a guide for self-medication. Patients should seek professional advice from qualified Chinese medicine practitioners.

Foreword

Since the late 20th century, Chinese medicine, including acupuncture and herbal medicine, has been increasingly used throughout the world. The parallel development and spread of evidence-based medicine has provided challenges and opportunities for Chinese medicine. The opportunities have been evidence-based medicine's emphasis on the effective use of the best available clinical evidence, incorporating the clinicians' clinical experience, subject to patients' preference. Such practices have a patient focus which reflects the historical nature of Chinese medicine practice. However, the challenges are also significant due to the fact that, despite the long term development and very rich literature accumulated over 2,000 years, there is an overall lack of high level clinical evidence for many of the interventions used in Chinese medicine.

To address this knowledge gap, we need to generate clinical evidence through high quality clinical studies and to evaluate evidence to enable effective use of such available evidence to promote evidence-based Chinese medicine practice.

Modern Chinese medicine is rooted in its classical literature and the legacies of ancient doctors, grounded in the practice of expert clinicians and increasingly informed by clinical and experimental research efforts. In recognition of the unique features of Chinese medicine, for each of the conditions in this series a "whole-evidence" approach is used to provide a synthesis of different types and levels of evidence to enable practitioners to make clinical decisions informed by the current best evidence.

There are four main components of this "whole-evidence" approach. Firstly, we present the current approaches to the diagnosis, differentiation and treatment of each condition based on expert consensus in published textbooks and clinical guidelines. This provides an overview of how the condition is currently managed. The second section provides an analysis of the condition in historical context based on systematic searches of the *Zhong Hua Yi Dian* 中华医典 which includes the full texts of more than 1,000 classical medical books. These analyses provide objective views on how the condition has been treated over two millennia, reveal continuities and discontinuities between traditional and modern practice, and suggest avenues for future research.

The third component is the assessment of evidence derived from modern clinical studies of Chinese medicine interventions. The methods established by the *Cochrane Collaboration* are used as the basis for conducting systematic reviews and undertaking meta-analyses of outcome data for randomised controlled trials (RCTs). In addition, the clinical relevance of meta-analysis data is enhanced by examining the herbal formulae, individual herbs and acupuncture treatments that were assessed in the RCTs and the evidence base is broadened by the inclusion of data from controlled clinical trials and non-controlled studies. The fourth component is to determine how the herbal medicine interventions may achieve the effects indicated by the clinical trials. Thus for each of the most frequently used herbs we provide reviews of their effects in pre-clinical models and their likely mechanisms of action.

For each condition, this "whole-evidence" approach links clinical expertise, historical precedent, clinical research data and experimental research to provide the reader with assessments of the current state of the evidence for the efficacy, effectiveness and safety of Chinese medicine interventions using herbal medicines, acupuncture and moxibustion and other health care practices such as *tai chi* 太极.

Since these books are available in Chinese and English, they can benefit patients, practitioners and educators internationally and enable practitioners to make clinical decisions informed by the current best evidence.

These publications represent a major milestone in the development of Chinese medicine and make a significant contribution to the development of evidence-based Chinese medicine globally.

Co-Editors-in-Chief

Distinguished Professor Charlie Changli Xue, RMIT University, Australia

Professor Chuanjian Lu, Guangdong Provincial Hospital of Chinese Medicine, China

Purpose of the Monograph

This book is intended for clinicians, researchers and educators. It can be used to inform tertiary education and clinical practice by providing systematic, multi-dimensional assessments of the best available evidence for using Chinese medicine to manage each common clinical condition.

How to Use This Monograph

Some Definitions

A glossary is included, containing terms and definitions which frequently appear in the book. It also describes the definitions of statistical tests, methodological terms, evaluation tools and interventions. For example, in this book, Integrative Medicine refers to the combined use of a Chinese medicine treatment with conventional medical management, and Combination Therapies refers to two or more Chinese medicines from different therapy groups (Chinese herbal medicine, acupuncture or other Chinese medicine therapies) administered together. Terminology used throughout the monograph is based on the World Health Organisation's *Standard Terminologies on Traditional Medicine in the Western Pacific Region* (2007) where possible or from the cited reference.

Data Analysis and Interpretation of Results

In order to synthesise the clinical evidence, a range of statistical analysis approaches are used. In general, the effect size for dichotomous data is reported as a risk ratio (RR) with 95% confidence intervals (CI), and for continuous data, they are reported as mean difference (MD) with 95% CI. Statistically significant effects are indicated with an asterisk (*). Readers should note that statistical significance does not necessarily correspond with a clinically important effect. Interpretation of results should take into consideration of the clinical significance, quality of studies (expressed as high, low or unclear risk of bias in this book) and heterogeneity amongst the studies. Tests for heterogeneity are conducted using the I^2 statistic. An I^2 score greater than 50% may indicate substantial heterogeneity.

Use of Evidence in Practice

The Grading of Recommendations Assessment, Development and Evaluation (GRADE) approach was used to summarise the results and certainty of the evidence for critical and important comparisons and outcomes. Due to the diverse nature of Chinese medicine practice, treatment recommendations are not included with the summary of findings tables. Therefore, readers will need to interpret the evidence with reference to the local practice environment.

Limitations

Readers should note some of the methodological limitations of the classical literature and the clinical evidence.

- Search terms used to search the *Zhong Hua Yi Dian* 中华医典 database may not include all terms that have been used for the condition, which may alter the findings.
- Chinese language has changed over time. Citations have been interpreted for analysis, and such interpretations may be subject to disagreement.
- Chinese medicine theory has evolved over time. As such, concepts described in classical Chinese medical literature may no longer be found in contemporary works.

- Symptoms described in citations may be common to many conditions, and a judgment was required to determine the likelihood of the citation being related to the condition. This may have introduced some bias due to the subjective nature of the judgment.
- The vast majority of the clinical evidence for Chinese medicine treatments has come from China. The applicability of the findings to other populations and other countries requires further assessment.
- Many studies included participants with varying disease severity. Where possible, subgroup analyses were undertaken to examine the effects in different sub-populations. As this was not always possible, the findings may be limited to the population included, and not to sub-populations.
- The potential risk of bias found in many included studies suggested methodological limitations. The findings for GRADE assessments based on studies of very low to moderate quality evidence should be interpreted accordingly.
- Nine major English and Chinese language databases were searched to identify clinical studies, in addition to clinical trial registers. Other studies may exist which were not identified through searches, and which may alter the findings.
- The calculation of frequency of herbal formula use was based on formula names. It is possible that studies evaluated herbal treatments with the same or similar herb ingredients, but which were given different formula names. Due to the complexity of herbal formulas, it was considered not appropriate to make a judgment as to the similarity of formulas for analysis. As such, the frequency of formulas reported in Chapter 5 may be underestimated.
- The most frequently utilised herbs which may have contributed to the treatment effect have been described in Chapter 5. These herbs may provide leads for further exploration. Calculation of the herbs with potential effect is based on frequency of formulae reported in the studies, and does not take into consideration the clinical implications and functions of every herb in a formula.

Authors and Contributors

CO-EDITORS-IN-CHIEF

Distinguished Prof. Charlie Changli Xue (*RMIT University, Australia*)
Prof. Chuanjian Lu (*Guangdong Provincial Hospital of Chinese Medicine, China*)

CO-DEPUTY EDITORS-IN-CHIEF

Assoc. Prof. Anthony Lin Zhang (*RMIT University, Australia*)
Dr. Brian H May (*RMIT University, Australia*)
Prof. Xinfeng Guo (*Guangdong Provincial Hospital of Chinese Medicine, China*)
Prof. Zehuai Wen (*Guangdong Provincial Hospital of Chinese Medicine, China*)

LEAD AUTHORS

Dr. Claire Shuiqing Zhang (*RMIT University, Australia*)
Dr. Dihui Zhang (*Guangdong Provincial Hospital of Chinese Medicine, China*)

CO-AUTHORS

RMIT University (Australia):
Dr. Mary Xinmei Zhang
Assoc. Prof. Anthony Lin Zhang
Distinguished Prof. Charlie Changli Xue

Guangdong Provincial Hospital of Chinese Medicine (China):

Prof. Chuanjian Lu
Prof. Dingkun Lin
Prof. Yongjin Li
Prof. Xinfeng Guo

Member of Advisory Committee and Panel

CO-CHAIRS OF PROJECT PLANNING COMMITTEE

Prof. Peter J Coloe (*RMIT University, Australia*)
Prof. Yubo Lyu (*Guangdong Provincial Hospital of Chinese Medicine, China*)
Prof. Dacan Chen (*Guangdong Provincial Hospital of Chinese Medicine, China*)

CENTRE ADVISORY COMMITTEE (ALPHABETICAL ORDER)

Prof. Keji Chen (*The Chinese Academy of Sciences, China*)
Prof. Aiping Lu (*Hong Kong Baptist University, China*)
Prof. Caroline Smith (*University of Western Sydney, Australia*)
Prof. David F Story (*RMIT University, Australia*)

METHODOLOGY EXPERT ADVISORY PANEL (ALPHABETICAL ORDER)

Prof. Zhaoxiang Bian (*Hong Kong Baptist University, China*)
The Late Prof. George Lewith (*University of Southampton, United Kingdom*)
Prof. Lixing Lao (*The University of Hong Kong, China*)
Prof. Jianping Liu (*Beijing University of Chinese Medicine, China*)
Prof. Frank Thien (*Monash University, Australia*)
Prof. Jialiang Wang (*Sichuan University, China*)

CONTENT EXPERT ADVISORY PANEL (ALPHABETICAL ORDER)

Prof. Fang Zeng (*Chengdu University of Chinese Medicine, Sichuan, China*)

Prof. Bin Li (*Beijing Hospital of Chinese Medicine, Beijing, China*)

Prof. Minshan Feng (*Wangjing Hospital of China Academy of Chinese Medical Sciences, Beijing, China*)

Prof. Mingsheng Tan (*China-Japan Friendship Hospital, Beijing, China*)

Distinguished Professor
Charlie Changli Xue, PhD

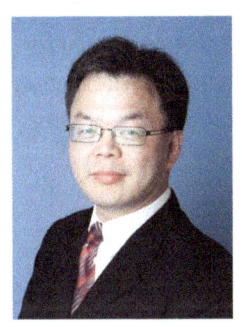

Distinguished Professor Charlie Changli Xue holds a Bachelor of Medicine (majoring in Chinese Medicine) from Guangzhou University of Chinese Medicine, China (1987) and a PhD from RMIT University, Australia (2000). He has been an academic, researcher, regulator and practitioner for almost three decades. Professor Xue has made significant contributions to evidence-based educational development, clinical research, regulatory framework and policy development and provision of high quality clinical care to the community. Professor Xue is recognised internationally as an expert in evidence-based traditional medicine and integrative healthcare.

Professor Xue is the Inaugural National Chair of the Chinese Medicine Board of Australia appointed by the Australian Health Workforce Ministerial Council (in 2011), and he was reappointed for a second term in 2014 and a third term in 2017. Since 2007, he has been a Member of the World Health Organization (WHO) Expert Advisory Panel for Traditional and Complementary Medicine, Geneva. Professor Xue is also Honorary Senior Principal Research Fellow at the Guangdong Provincial Academy of Chinese Medical Sciences, China.

At RMIT, Professor Xue is Executive Dean, School of Health and Biomedical Sciences. He is also Director, World Health Organization (WHO) Collaborating Centre for Traditional Medicine.

Between 1995 and 2010, Professor Xue was Discipline Head of Chinese Medicine at RMIT University. He leads the development of five successful undergraduate and postgraduate degree programs in Chinese Medicine at RMIT University which is now a global leader in Chinese medicine education and research.

Professor Xue's research has been supported by over AU$15 million research grants including six project grants from the Australian Government's National Health & Medical Research Council (NHMRC) and two Australian Research Council (ARC) grants. He has contributed over 200 publications and has been frequently invited as keynote speaker for numerous national and international conferences. Professor Xue has contributed to over 300 media interviews on issues related to complementary medicine education, research, regulation and practice.

Professor Chuanjian Lu, MD

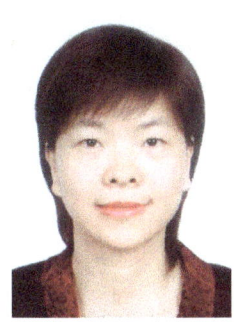 Professor Chuanjian Lu, Doctor of Medicine. She is the vice president of Guangdong Provincial Hospital of Chinese Medicine (Guangdong Provincial Academy of Chinese Medical Sciences, Second Clinical Medical College of Guangzhou University of Chinese Medicine). She also is the chair of the Guangdong Traditional Chinese Medicine (TCM) Standardization Technical Committee, and the vice-chair of the Immunity Specialty Committee of the World Federation of Chinese Medicine Societies (WFCMS).

Professor Lu has engaged in scientific research into TCM, clinical practice and teaching for some 25 years. Her research has been devoted to integrated traditional and Western medicine. She has edited and published 12 monographs and 120 academic research articles as first author and corresponding author with over 30 articles being included in SCI journals. She has received widespread recognition for her achievements with awards for "Excellent Teacher of South China", "National Outstanding Women TCM Doctor", and "National Outstanding Young Doctor of TCM". She also received "The Science and Technology Star of the Association of Chinese Medicine", the "National Excellent Science and Technology Workers of China Award" and the "Five-Continent Women's Scientific Awards of China Medical Women's Association".

Professor Lu has won the Award of Science and Technology Progress over 10 times from Guangdong Provincial Government, China Association of Chinese Medicine and Chinese Hospital Association.

Acknowledgements

The authors and contributors would like to acknowledge the valuable contributions of the following people who assisted with database searches, data extraction, data screening, data assessment, translation of documents, editing, and/or administrative tasks: Ms. Mary-Jo O'Rourke AE, Mr. Yu Huo, Ms. Jingmin Xiao, Mr. Jinhao Lin, Mr. Yanjun Chen, Mr. Jiheng Zhan, Mr. Fangjun Xiao, Mr. Tiancheng Deng.

Contents

Contents

Contents

Contents

List of Figures

List of Tables

1

Introduction to Cervical Radiculopathy

OVERVIEW

Cervical radiculopathy is a cervical degenerative disc disease that results in neck and arm pain radiating to the upper extremities and may generate progressive neurological sensory deficits. Cervical radiculopathy can significantly reduce the quality of life. This chapter reviews the definition, epidemiology, pathological processes, diagnostic procedures, management and prognosis of cervical radiculopathy.

Definition of Cervical Radiculopathy

Cervical radiculopathy (CR) is a neurological dysfunction characterised by radicular pain in the upper limbs.[1] It is typically associated with inflammation in the nerve root and/or limited cervical nerve root canal space generated by disc herniation or degenerative disorders of the zygapophysial joints.[2] The North American Spine Society (NASS) defines CR as *"pain in a radicular pattern in one or both upper extremities related to compression and/or irritation of one or more cervical nerve roots. Frequent signs and symptoms include varying degrees of sensory, motor, and reflex changes as well as dysesthesias and paraesthesias related to nerve roots without evidence of spinal cord dysfunction (myelopathy)".*[3] Age, gender, ethnicity and high-risk occupation have been found to be factors associated with CR.[4–6]

Clinical Presentation of Cervical Radiculopathy

Typical clinical manifestations of CR include neck pain, unilateral or bilateral radiating arm pain, paraesthesia, sensory or motor deficits and reflex impairment or loss in the upper extremities and neck.[2,3,7] Symptoms of CR usually present in a dermatome pattern according to the compression of different levels of nerve roots. Table 1.1 summarises the different patterns of CR based on the affected nerve roots.

Symptoms related to CR, especially neck pain, commonly present unilaterally.[7,8] In some cases, when both sides of the nerve root are irritated by severe osteophytes at one cervical level, CR symptoms can also manifest bilaterally.[8] Physical activities such as extension or rotation to the affected limb can aggravate the symptoms by decreasing the neural foramen space, while abducting movements may alleviate CR symptoms.[7] In clinical practice, CR is usually characterised by radicular upper extremity pain.[2,3] However, it should be noted that the presentation of pain can be limited to the

Table 1.1. Patterns of Cervical Radiculopathy

Nerve Root	Pain Distribution	Motor Dysfunction	Sensory Dysfunction	Reflex Impairment
C4	Lower neck and trapezius	Shoulder elevation	Cape distribution	NA
C5	Neck, shoulder, lateral and arm	Deltoid, elbow flexion and shoulder abduction	Lateral arm	Biceps
C6	Neck, radial arm and thumb	Biceps and elbow flexion/wrist extension	Radial forearm and thumb	Brachioradialis
C7	Neck, dorsal forearm and long fingers	Triceps and elbow extension/wrist flexion	Dorsal forearm and long finger	Triceps
C8	Neck, medial forearm and ulnar digits	Thumb extension	Medial forearm and ulnar digits	NA

Adapted from Corey *et al.* and Buxton *et al.*[7,8]
Abbreviations: C, cervical segment; NA, not applicable.

shoulder without a radiating pattern. Some patients with CR may only manifest sensory or motor deficits symptoms without complaining of pain.[7]

Epidemiology

Cervical radiculopathy can be acquired by people of any age group and the prevalence rate has been identified to peak at the age of around 50 years.[5,8,9] The Global Burden of Diseases, Injuries, and Risk Factors Study 2017 (GBD 2017) published results of global, regional and national epidemiological research in 195 countries, indicating that the prevalence of neck pain in 2017 was more than 288 million globally, with an age standardised point prevalence per 100,000 population of 3,551.1 (95% uncertainty interval 3,139.5 to 3,977.9).[10,11] In the regional level, the highest age standardised point prevalence of neck pain per 100,000 population in 2017 were in western Europe (4,636.1 (95% uncertainty interval 4,077.2 to 5,250.5)), East Asia (4,589.7 (95% uncertainty interval 4,042.7 to 5,168.9)), and North Africa and the Middle East (4,458.4 (95% uncertainty interval 3,917.7 to 5,022.4)).[10,11] While on the national level, China is one of the countries in which the highest rates of age standardises annual incidence of neck pain being observed in 2017 (1,037.7 (95% uncertainty interval 917.3 to 1,176.9)).[10,11]

Although the age standardised point prevalence and annual incidence of neck pain have not changed over the past three decades in general, a statistically significant increase in the age standardised point prevalence of neck pain was found in some regions including western Europe, southern sub-Saharan Africa and eastern sub-Saharan Africa between 1990 and 2017.[10,11] Whereas the neck pain data was not specific for CR, the increasing trend in the prevalence of neck pain from 1990 to 2017 may raise public health concern about CR.[10] As for the specific prevalence of CR, a recently published cross-sectional community-based study indicated that the prevalence of CR was 13.76% in 3,859 observations in China.[4] The specific prevalence information of CR in Australia is lacking.

Burden

The GBD 2017 study also pointed out that neck pain, being one of the major complaints in CR, was the fourth greatest cause for Years Lived with Disability (YLDs).[10] The global YLDs caused by neck pain was more than 28.6 million, with an increase of 44.4% from 1990 to 2017.[10] Based on the Cost of Pain in Australia, it is estimated that there were 112,000 Disability-Adjusted Life Years (DALYs) due to neck pain in Australia in 2016.[12] The economic burden of general neck pain was found to be high according to the clinical practice guideline of the American Physical Therapy Association. It can lead to high expenses for medical management and compensation expenditures for patients.[13] Neck pain was identified as the second annual compensation cost in the United States (US).[14] Nygren *et al.* reported that neck and shoulder disorders contributed 18% to the total annual disability payments.[15]

In terms of the cost for CR management, there was no direct economic burden of non-surgical management of CR from data identified in the database search. A review of the cost-effectiveness of surgery for unilateral CR in the US military showed that the total cost of posterior cervical foraminotomy (PCF) was as high as US$20,094. The cost of anterior cervical discectomy and fusion (ACDF) was even higher, reaching US$30,553.[16]

Risk Factors

Age, gender, ethnicity and high-risk occupation have been found to be factors associated with CR.

Age

Advancing age is considered one of the main risk factors in the process of disc degeneration.[17] Early epidemiological research by Radhakrishnan *et al.* identified that the incidence of CR was age-specific, peaking at 58.3 per 100,000 people per year in the 50–54 years age group and then decreasing sharply in the 60+ years age group.[5] Similar findings were also reported in a later military survey (incidence peaked at age 40 years) and two investigations in China (incidence peaked at 50 years and 60 years, respectively).[4,6,9] It was suggested that the ageing process gradually mitigates the inflammatory effect of the nucleus, which contributes to a lower risk of CR.[9]

Gender

It seems that CR is more prevalent in females than in males. Recent epidemiological investigations have found higher incidence rates in females.[4,6,9,18] The GBD 2017 study also reported that general neck pain in 2017 was higher in females compared with males, although this was not significant at the 0.05 level.[10,11] As a result, the global point prevalence of neck pain in 2017 ranked as the 9th cause of YLDs in females and the 11th cause in males.[10,11]

The reason for this remains unclear. Sex-related biomechanical properties such as discoligamentous structures in the cervical spine, sex hormones or lifestyle could be possible factors but need further confirmation.[6] Lv *et al.* (2018) also found that menopause is a factor associated with cervical spondylosis.[4]

Ethnicity

An epidemiological review of the US military's database from 2000 to 2009 reported that among the 24,742 individuals who were diagnosed with cervical radiculopathy with an incidence of 1.79 per 1,000 person-years, white people have a higher risk of acquiring CR (unadjusted IR: 1.93 per thousand person-years) than those of African and other ethnicities (unadjusted IR: 1.54 and 1.43 per thousand person-years, respectively).[6]

Occupation

Several studies have shown that heavy manual labour is a risk factor for degenerative cervical spine disorders.[6,18–20] A large-sized epidemiological research on the US military found that people working in senior military positions and/or in the Army or Air Force had a higher risk of acquiring CR, as these careers involved heavy labour and vigorous physical activity.[6]

Pathological Processes

Cervical radiculopathy involves pathological processes such as mechanical compression, neuropraxia and inflammation of the cervical root and/or roots at or near the cervical neural foramen.[1,21] Two common pathologies including cervical disc degeneration and cervical spondylosis have been identified to generate CR.[1,21,22] Spinal tumours, injuries with avulsion of the nerve root, infections, twisted vertebral arteries, synovial or meningeal cysts, and dural arteriovenous fistulae have also been found to induce CR by decreasing the space for cervical roots, but are not commonly seen in clinical observation.[21,23–25] In epidemiological research by Radhakrishnan *et al.*, 20–25% of CR cases were generated by cervical disc degeneration, while 70–75% were associated with cervical spondylosis.[5]

Cervical Disc Degeneration

In a critical review of the pathophysiology of disc degeneration by Hadjipavlou *et al.*, several factors other than ageing have been shown to be related to disc degeneration. These include genetic factors, nutrition, toxic factors (e.g., nicotine), metabolic disorders, low-grade infection, neurogenic inflammation, autoimmune issues and mechanical factors.[17] The authors indicated that the ageing process is the primary factor according to epidemiological and laboratory evidence.

The process of cervical disc degeneration starts at the age of 20 years in humans.[26] In the ageing process, glycosaminoglycan proteins, which are the basic structure of the nucleus pulposus, gradually decrease in size and number. As the main function of the glycosaminoglycan proteins is attracting water molecules, loss of the water content of the intervertebral disc occurs progressively with ageing, causing the nucleus pulposus to become a blurred fibrocartilaginous mass.[26,27] Changes in the nucleus pulposus and part of the outer annulus fibrosus cause the cervical disc to become more easily compressed and less elastic with advancing age, and consequently lead to disc height loss and herniation progressively into the spinal canal and posterolaterally into the neural foramen.[27] A compressive herniated disc can cause nerve root or cord impingement, generating upper extremity pain, and sensory and motor deficits.[28] Laboratory evidence also showed that a herniated cervical disc spontaneously releases inflammatory cytokines including interleukin (IL)-6, IL-8, nitric oxide, tumour necrosis factor and prostaglandin E2, which contribute to radiculopathy pain.[29]

Degenerative Cervical Spondylosis

Degenerative cervical spondylosis of the zygapophysial and uncovertebral joints (Luschka joint) begins around ten years after the start of the cervical disc degeneration process, resulting from mechanical incompetence of the cervical motion segment.[22,30] When disc height loss occurs, the zygapophysial and uncovertebral joints come into contact and overlap, which causes the formation of osteophytes as a self-protection mechanism. The protrusions of osteophytes then induce cervical stenosis and compress the nerve, generating CR.[30,31]

Diagnosis

A diagnosis of CR is based on patients' symptoms, physical diagnostic tests and medical imaging confirmation.[2,3] Bono *et al.* in the NASS guideline synthesised the clinical evidence for the diagnosis methods for CR with GRADE recommendations (Table 1.2).[3]

Medical History

Typical presentations including upper extremity pain (with/without a radiating pattern), motor or sensory deficits and abnormal tendon reflexes are commonly seen in CR patients. Atypical manifestations such as shoulder or hand muscle weakness, chest or deep breast pain

Table 1.2. **Diagnosis Methods for Cervical Radiculopathy**[3,7]

Diagnosis Method	Details	GRADE Recommendation[3]
Patient's history and symptoms	Common findings: Arm pain, neck pain, scapular or periscapular pain, paraesthesias, numbness and sensory changes, weakness or abnormal deep tendon reflexes in the arm.	Level B
	Atypical findings: Deltoid weakness, scapular winging, weakness of the intrinsic muscles of the hand, chest or deep breast pain, and headaches.	Level B
Physical diagnostic tests	Upper extremity neurological examination including motor tests for weakness and sensory tests for all dermatomes, and reflex tests.	Level B
	Provocative tests including the Spurling test and shoulder abduction signs.	Level B
Medical diagnostic imaging techniques	Magnetic resonance imaging	Level B
	Computed tomography	Level B
	Computed tomography myelography	Level B
Electrodiagnostics tests	Electromyography	Level I (insufficient evidence)

and headaches can also be considered in the diagnosis of CR.[3] The type and dermatome distribution of CR symptoms are determined by the nerve root compression located at different cervical levels.[7,8,21] In performing diagnosis, health practitioners can refer to the characteristic presentations in order to locate the affected nerve root (Table 1.1). In general, the C7 nerve root is the most commonly affected, while the C6 nerve root is the second most commonly involved.[7,21]

Provocative Tests

According to the NASS guideline, provocative tests can be considered in CR diagnosis.[3] The Spurling test, which can provoke arm pain in the

CR patient by exacerbating the encroachment on the cervical nerve roots by intentionally narrowing the neural foramen, has been widely adopted in the clinical diagnosis process.[7,21,22] It can be performed by asking the patient to extend their neck and rotate their head to the affected body side, then applying a downward load on their head.[7,21,22] The Spurling test was considered a specific but not sensitive test for CR in previous reviews and guidelines.[3,21,22] In a recent study, the Spurling test showed 95% sensitivity and 94% specificity in detecting CR, as confirmed by computerised tomography (CT) and magnetic resonance imaging (MRI).[32] Thoomes *et al.* systematically reviewed the evidence for the Spurling test in diagnosing CR and indicated that this test was moderate in sensitivity and high in specificity.[33]

In contrast, the shoulder abduction test is considered to alleviate CR symptoms by expanding the intervertebral foramen. This manoeuvre is performed by raising the patient's arm above their head.[22] Current evidence showed moderate sensitivity and high specificity of this test.[33]

Thoomes *et al.* also introduced an "arm squeeze test" of high sensitivity and specificity for CR diagnosis.[33] To perform this test, the examiner stands behind the patient, then squeezes the middle third of the patient's upper arm with the thumb from the posterior (on the triceps) and the other fingers from the anterior (on the biceps). The test is positive if the patient reports a Visual Analogue Scale (VAS) score of 3 or greater when the examiner squeezes with moderate compression.

Other provocative tests were also evaluated by Thoomes *et al.* in their systematic review, such as the upper limb neural tension test and the traction test. The authors recommended that a combination of a positive Spurling test, axial traction test and arm squeeze test can be used to diagnose CR when consistent with the clinical presentation and other physical examinations.[33]

Table 1.3 summarises the evidence strength for the provocative tests in the systematic review by Thoomes *et al.*[33]

Medical Imaging

Medical imaging for the diagnosis of CR can provide anterior, posterior and lateral views of the cervical spine.[34] Degenerative changes,

Table 1.3. Provocative Tests for Diagnosis of Cervical Radiculopathy[33]

Provocative Test	Sensitivity	Specificity
Spurling test	Moderate	High
Upper limb neural tension tests (ULNTs, ULNT1, ULNT2a and 2b)	Combination of four ULNTs: High ULNT1: High	ULNT3: High
Shoulder abduction test	Moderate	High
Traction test	Low	High
Arm Squeeze test	High	High

Abbreviation: ULNT, upper limb neural tension tests.

formation of osteophytes and neuroforaminal narrowing that generate CR symptoms can be observed and evaluated via medical imaging.[7,34] MRI and CT scans are the two most frequently used diagnostic techniques for CR.[3]

In the NASS guideline, an MRI scan is recommended for confirming the correlative compressive lesions including cervical herniation and spondylosis for CR patients without satisfactory conservative treatment and when preparing for interventional or surgical treatment.[3] Findings from MRI scans should be correlated with clinical presentations because of the high false-positive and false-negative rates.[7] For patients who have contraindications for MRI, such as those who have metallic implants or cardiac pacemakers, should be considered for CT examination.[3] CT myelography is also recommended for further evaluation where MRI findings are inconsistent with the patient's clinical presentation.[3]

Electromyography

Electromyography (EMG) is considered to provide useful evidence for differentiating peripheral nerve entrapment syndromes (e.g., carpal or cubital tunnel syndromes) from CR.[7,34,35] However, due to insufficient clinical evidence, the NASS guideline does not draw a conclusion in the recommended level of EMG for CR.[3]

Management

A series of management strategies for CR has been developed in clinical practice. Roth *et al.* and Corey *et al.* summarised that the preliminary management goals in CR are to minimise pain, improve neurological function and prevent recurrence.[7,22] Pharmacotherapies, surgical interventions and physiotherapy are commonly introduced by contemporary clinical reviews and guidelines for CR.[1–3,8,36] At least three evidence-based clinical practice guidelines have been published that detail clinical management of CR.[2,3,36] The NASS evidence-based guideline by Bono *et al.*[3] provides recommendations on clinical questions on the definition, diagnosis and management of CR. The Danish Health Authority guideline by Kjaer *et al.* summarises the contemporary non-surgical evidence and recommendations on CR[2] while Latka *et al.* from the Polish Society of Spinal Surgery developed a surgical treatment recommendation guideline for CR.[36]

Pharmacotherapy

Pharmaceutical medications are commonly mentioned or recommended in managing CR in contemporary reviews or guidelines.[2,3,7,22,35] However, due to insufficient CR clinical trial evidence, the NASS guideline states that the role of pharmacotherapy remains unclear in the management of CR.[3] In general, there are three categories of pharmacotherapy options for CR according to current guidelines and reviews.

Nonsteroidal Anti-Inflammatory Medication

Nonsteroidal anti-inflammatory drugs (NSAIDs) are traditionally considered the first-line medications for CR.[22] NSAIDs can inhibit the activity of cyclooxygenase enzymes to reduce the prostaglandin level in humans, which may alleviate the inflammation in both herniated and degenerated discs.[22,29] In the acute stage of CR, Corey *et al.* (2014) recommended a two-week trial NSAID management at a therapeutic dose to relieve symptoms.[7] In the Danish guideline, the work groups recommended that the use of oral NSAIDs should follow the general Danish guideline for pain and the use of NSAIDs:[2]

- Paracetamol, maximum dose 1 g * 4 doses;
- In cases of suspected inflammatory response: COX inhibitors, e.g., ibuprofen 200–400 mg * 3 doses or naproxen 250–500 mg * 2 doses; and
- The NSAID treatment should not last more than 4–8 weeks and it is important to follow up and re-examine the treatment effect.

In a more recent Danish guideline, the specialist and expert work groups recommended NSAIDs and tramadol as second-line drugs that should be used after careful consideration.[2] Topical NSAID treatment was evaluated in one study by comparing a diclofenac gel with a placebo gel for CR. Although the diclofenac gel achieved a more positive outcome than the placebo gel, the high risk of bias limited its evidence strength according to the Danish guideline.

Steroids

Oral steroid therapy has not been recommended in either the NASS or Danish guidelines; however, some general reviews have suggested it could be optional management for CR.[7,22,35,37] Steroids have a strong anti-inflammatory function and they are considered to have an analgesic effect by inhibiting the perineural inflammatory mediators of herniated discs.[29,35] Although oral steroids are often selected for managing acute radicular pain, high-quality supporting evidence remains lacking.[7,37] Long-term oral use of steroids may lead to a series of known adverse effects.[7] Corey *et al.* also stated that the clinical efficacy of oral steroids can be an indicator for further corticosteroid injection treatment.[7] Ghasemi *et al.* conducted a short course oral prednisolone randomised clinical trial (RCT), recruiting 60 CR participants in acute phases. The study showed significant analgesic efficacy of prednisolone compared with a placebo in a short-term observation period.[38]

Epidural steroid injection (ESI) therapy is usually practised via transforaminal or interlaminar approaches. Similar to oral steroid treatment, ESI is intended to reduce the inflammation of the affected nerve root, but by directly infiltrating the nerve root with steroids.[39] ESI can be considered for patients with persistent radicular symptoms after four to six weeks of conservative treatment.[37] In the NASS guideline, ESI treatment is considered a GRADE C Level recommendation with limited high-quality evidence.[3] A more recent study systematically reviewed the long-term analgesic effect of cervical epidural injections for neck and upper extremity pain due to cervical disc herniation. The authors synthesised studies with level 2 evidence.[40] One high-quality RCT was included, showing that interlaminar epidural injections with or without steroids were effective for participants in the long term.[41] As severe complications such as spinal cord injury and even death have been reported when performing ESI, the NASS guideline recommends that fluoroscopic or CT guidance should be considered when using this approach.[3,42,43]

Opioid Medication

Tramadol, an opioid medication, was recommended by Roth *et al.* for managing severe pain in acute and sub-acute CR.[22] It can provide neuropathic pain alleviation.[44] However, due to insufficient clinical evidence and significant side effects, the Danish guideline indicates that tramadol should not be preferred over NSAID medications.[2]

Non-Pharmacological Interventions

Patient Education and Advice

The Danish guideline recommends the provision of structured and individualised education to CR patients about its anatomical and physiological basis, pain mechanisms, disease prognosis and guidance on appropriate physical activities. The expert group indicated that patient education and professional advice provided along with reassurance to CR patients can help them to understand their condition better, which is beneficial for the management process.[2]

Manipulation Treatment

Manipulation therapy is defined as "skilled hand movements" provided by health professionals including physiotherapists, chiropractors and osteopaths.[45] It is believed to be beneficial for improving tissue extensibility, relaxing muscles and alleviating pain and soft-tissue swelling and inflammation.[46] In the Danish guideline, spinal manipulation therapy is recommended in combination with patient education and advice on pain management and physical activity.[2] The practice is recommended to start at low intensity and gradually strengthen according to the patient's condition and preference. A recent multi-centre RCT (level 2 evidence) showed that thoracic spine manipulation had better results in relation to pain relief, disability, cervical range of motion improvement and deep neck flexor endurance in the short term compared with placebo manipulation.[47] In the NASS guideline, the expert group indicated that severe complications may present, based on previous case reports, and recommends pre-manipulation imaging to reduce the risks before treatment.[3]

Exercise Therapy

Motor control exercises, which consist of a set of specific exercises to train deep cervical muscles without aggravating pain, are evaluated in the Danish guideline.[2] Clinical evidence showed benefits in short-term pain relief, but was limited by the study quality. Motor control exercises were recommended for patients with recent onset of CR combined with other therapies in this guideline.[2] A recent RCT conducted a three-month-long neck-specific training in 72 participants in comparison with prescribed physical activity. The result showed that both exercise therapies demonstrated long-term benefits in pain management, disability and quality of life.[48]

Directional exercise is also recommended for managing CR by the Danish guideline.[2] Although no clinical evidence is identified, the expert working group indicated that a specific maximum-range neck movement performed in both directions can be beneficial in alleviating radiating pain with low risk of harm. However, this exercise needs the patient's full understanding and adjustment of the exercise to perform this approach.[2]

Mechanical Traction

Mechanical traction is a pulling force approach for the cervical spine using a mechanical system, which can be applied temporarily or continuously. Traction treatment has the function of separating the vertebral bodies, expanding the intervertebral foramen and decreasing the compression of the nerve roots.[49] Considering the low quality of clinical evidence and the potential mild harm for CR patients, the Danish guideline indicates that mechanical traction should be selected as an adjunct therapy integrated with other physiotherapy treatments.[2]

Surgery

In the NASS guideline, operative treatment can provide rapid CR symptom relief compared with conservative treatment.[3] Woods *et al.* pointed out that up to 25% of patients with cervical radiculopathy had persistent symptoms and required surgical intervention.[1] For cervical radiculopathy in the absence of myelopathy, surgery is recommended in patients who have root-related dysfunction (pain, sensory disturbance, weakness) for at least six weeks, have concordant root compression in advanced imaging and have undergone failed non-surgical treatments.[1] For those experiencing significant or progressive motor deficits, decompression surgery can also be considered even when the disease course is less than six weeks.[1]

In clinical practice, surgical approaches via anterior or posterior directions have been developed in managing CR. The ACDF approach has been widely considered the "gold standard" for CR management at single or multiple levels (≤3) for its well-reported efficacy.[1,36] The NASS guideline conducted an evidence-based comparison between different surgical approaches (Table 1.4).

Table 1.4. Comparison of Different Surgical Treatments for Cervical Radiculopathy in North American Spine Society Guideline[3]

Comparison	Outcome	GRADE Recommendation
ACDF *vs.* ACD	An interbody graft for fusion is recommended to improve sagittal alignment in single-level CR after ACD.	Level B
ACDF with instrumentation *vs.* ACDF only	A cervical plate is suggested to improve sagittal alignment in single-level CR after ACDF.	Level B
	There is insufficient clinical evidence for multilevel ACDF comparison.	Work Group Consensus Statement
Anterior surgery *vs.* posterior surgery	Both ACDF and posterior foraminotomy are recommended for single-level CR secondary to disc herniation.	Level B
	ACDF is recommended for single-level CR when compared with a posterior approach.	Work Group Consensus Statement
Posterior decompression with fusion *vs.* posterior decompression only	Insufficient comparable data.	No evidence
ACDF and reconstruction with total disc replacement *vs.* ACDF only	Similar successful short-term outcome as for single-level CR.	Level B

Abbreviations: ACD, anterior cervical decompression; ACDF, anterior cervical decompression with fusion; CR, cervical radiculopathy; *vs.*, *versus*.

Long-term results (more than four years) of the surgical treatments are also discussed in the NASS guideline. This evidence-based clinical guideline showed benefits of surgical treatment in producing and maintaining long-term efficacy in managing CR.[3] In the more recent Polish surgical guideline for CR, surgical treatment was found to be effective in both medium- and long-term observations according to quantitative analysis.[36]

Although the clinical efficacy of surgical treatments for CR has been well established, the complications related to surgery cannot be ignored. For example, cases of specific graft-related complications, hardware failure, risk of pseudoarthrosis and adjacent segment degeneration after ACDF surgery have been reported in several studies.[50–52]

Limitations of Conventional Therapy

As stated above, the current conventional therapies are associated with certain limitations: e.g., the role of pharmacotherapy remains unclear in the management of CR; surgical treatments are proved effective but the complications related to surgery are of concern; manipulation treatment and mechanical traction are not considered as risk-free therapies. Therefore, clinical practice may consider incorporating other therapies, such as complementary and alternative therapies, if sufficient evidence supports their effectiveness and safety.

Prognosis

The clinical course of CR is expected to be long. A systematic review of the course of CR resulting from cervical disc herniation showed that substantial improvement was seen within four to six months from the onset of symptoms. The time to recovery was estimated to be from 24 to 36 months in most patients.[53]

The clinical course and prognostic models for conservative management, including physiotherapy and pharmacotherapy for CR, were evaluated in a prospective cohort study.[54] The researchers indicated that the clinical course of CR appeared to be long, with a recovery rate of only around 58% after one year. Less favourable prognoses were found in patients experiencing a longer course of symptoms, absence of paresthaesia, higher intensity neck pain and higher disability score at baseline and lower active rotation towards the affected side.[54]

Short-term outcomes of physiotherapy in the management of CR were reported by Cleland *et al.*[55] In a 28-day observation period, a series of predictive factors were found to have a positive outcome:

- Age of less than 54 years;
- Dominant arm not affected;
- Symptoms not exacerbated by looking down;
- Multimodal treatment (manipulation treatment, mechanical traction and deep neck flex or muscle strengthening) for at least 50% of the visits.

If any three of these factors were present, the probability of a short-term successful outcome was estimated to be 85% and increased to 90% if all the above four factors appeared.

In a long-term follow-up of patients undergoing posterior cervical foraminotomy, health-related quality of life was improved during a ten-year period.[56]

A summary of this chapter is presented in Table 1.5.

Table 1.5. Summary of Chapter 1

Definition	Cervical radiculopathy is a cervical degenerative disc disease manifesting radicular pain in the upper extremities.
Main characteristics	Typical characteristics of CR include neck pain, unilateral or bilateral radiating arm pain, sensory or motor dysfunction, and reflex impairment of the upper extremities.
Diagnosis	Patient's history and symptoms; Physical diagnostic tests; Medical diagnostic imaging: CT and MRI; and Electrodiagnostic tests.
Management	Pharmaceutical medications: NSAIDs, steroids and opioid medications; Physiotherapy: Patient education, manipulation treatment, exercise therapy and mechanical traction; and Surgery: Anterior and posterior approaches.

Abbreviations: CR, cervical radiculopathy; CT, computerised tomography; MRI, magnetic resonance imaging; NSAID, non-steroidal anti-inflammatory drug.

References

1. Woods BI, Hilibrand AS. (2015) Cervical radiculopathy: Epidemiology, etiology, diagnosis, and treatment. *J Spinal Disord Tech* **28**(5): E251–E259.
2. Kjaer P, Kongsted A, Hartvigsen J, *et al*. (2017) National clinical guidelines for non-surgical treatment of patients with recent onset neck pain or cervical radiculopathy. *Eur Spine J* **26**(9): 2242–2257.
3. Bono CM, Ghiselli G, Gilbert TJ, *et al*. (2011) An evidence-based clinical guideline for the diagnosis and treatment of cervical radiculopathy from degenerative disorders. *Spine J* **11**(1): 64–72.
4. Lv Y, Tian W, Chen D, *et al*. (2018) The prevalence and associated factors of symptomatic cervical spondylosis in Chinese adults: A community-based cross-sectional study. *BMC Musculoskelet Disord* **19**(1): 325.
5. Radhakrishnan K, Litchy WJ, O'Fallon WM, Kurland LT. (1994) Epidemiology of cervical radiculopathy: A population-based study from Rochester, Minnesota, 1976 through 1990. *Brain* **117**(Pt 2): 325–335.
6. Schoenfeld AJ, George AA, Bader JO, Caram PM, Jr. (2012) Incidence and epidemiology of cervical radiculopathy in the United States military: 2000 to 2009. *J Spinal Disord Tech* **25**(1): 17–22.
7. Corey DL, Comeau D. (2014) Cervical radiculopathy. *Med Clin North Am* **98**(4): 791–799, xii.
8. Buxton S, Vermeersch J, Dartevelle S. Cervical radiculopathy [cited 1 Oct 2019]. Available from: www.physio-pedia.com/Cervical_Radiculopathy#cite_note-Eubanks.2CJD-2.
9. Wang C, Tian F, Zhou Y, *et al*. (2016) The incidence of cervical spondylosis decreases with aging in the elderly, and increases with aging in the young and adult population: A hospital-based clinical analysis. *Clin Interv Aging* **11**: 47–53.
10. GBD (2017) Disease and Injury Incidence and Prevalence Collaborators. (2018) Global, regional, and national incidence, prevalence, and years lived with disability for 354 diseases and injuries for 195 countries and territories, 1990–2017: A systematic analysis for the Global Burden of Disease Study 2017. *Lancet* **392**(10159): 1789–1858.
11. Safiri S, Kolahi AA, Hoy D, *et al*. (2020) Global, regional, and national burden of neck pain in the general population, 1990–2017: Systematic analysis of the Global Burden of Disease Study 2017. *BMJ* **368**: m791.

12. Deloitte Access Economics. (2019) The cost of pain in Australia. Available from: https://www.painaustralia.org.au/static/uploads/files/the-cost-of-pain-in-australia-final-report-12mar-wfxbrfyboams.pdf.

13. Childs JD, Cleland JA, Elliott JM, *et al.* (2008) Neck pain: Clinical practice guidelines linked to the international classification of functioning, disability, and health from the orthopedic section of the American Physical Therapy Association. *J Orthop Sports Phys Ther* **38**(9): A1–A34.

14. Wright A, Mayer TG, Gatchel RJ. (1999) Outcomes of disabling cervical spine disorders in compensation injuries: A prospective comparison to tertiary rehabilitation response for chronic lumbar spinal disorders. *Spine* **24**(2): 178–183.

15. Nygren A, Berglund A, von Koch M. (1995) Neck-and-shoulder pain, an increasing problem: Strategies for using insurance material to follow trends. *Scand J Rehabil Med Suppl* **32**: 107–112.

16. Tumialan LM, Ponton RP, Gluf WM. (2010) Management of unilateral cervical radiculopathy in the military: The cost effectiveness of posterior cervical foraminotomy compared with anterior cervical discectomy and fusion. *Neurosurg Focus* **28**(5): E17.

17. Hadjipavlou AG, Tzermiadianos MN, Bogduk N, Zindrick MR. (2008) The pathophysiology of disc degeneration: A critical review. *J Bone Joint Surg Br* **90**(10): 1261–1270.

18. Singh S, Kumar D, Kumar S. (2014) Risk factors in cervical spondylosis. *J Clin Orthop Trauma* **5**(4): 221–226.

19. Mahbub MH, Laskar MS, Seikh FA, *et al.* (2006) Prevalence of cervical spondylosis and musculoskeletal symptoms among coolies in a city of Bangladesh. *J Occup Health* **48**(1): 69–73.

20. Takamiya Y, Nagata K, Fukuda K, *et al.* (2006) Cervical spine disorders in farm workers requiring neck extension actions. *J Orthop Sci* **11**(3): 235–240.

21. Abbed KM, Coumans JV. (2007) Cervical radiculopathy: Pathophysiology, presentation, and clinical evaluation. *Neurosurgery* **60**(1 Suppl 1): S28–S34.

22. Roth D, Mukai A, Thomas P, Hudgins TH, Alleva JT. (2009) Cervical radiculopathy. *Dis Mon* **55**(12): 737–756.

23. Horgan MA, Hsu FP, Frank EH. (1998) Cervical radiculopathy secondary to a tortuous vertebral artery. Case illustration. *J Neurosurg* **89**(3): 489.

24. Kohno M, Takahashi H, Ide K, Ishijima B, Yamada K, Nemoto S. (1996) A cervical dural arteriovenous fistula in a patient presenting with radiculopathy. Case report. *J Neurosurg* **84**(1): 119–123.

25. Shelerud RA, Paynter KS. (2002) Rarer causes of radiculopathy: Spinal tumors, infections, and other unusual causes. *Phys Med Rehabil Clin N Am* **13**(3): 645–696.

26. Oda J, Tanaka H, Tsuzuki N. (1988) Intervertebral disc changes with aging of human cervical vertebra: From the neonate to the eighties. *Spine* **13**(11): 1205–1211.

27. Blumenkrantz N, Sylvest J, Asboe-Hansen G. (1977) Local low-collagen content may allow herniation of intervertebral disc: Biochemical studies. *Biochem Med* **18**(3): 283–290.

28. Lestini WF, Wiesel SW. (1989) The pathogenesis of cervical spondylosis. *Clin Orthop Relat Res* **239**: 69–93.

29. Kang JD, Georgescu HI, McIntyre-Larkin L, Stefanovic-Racic M, Evans CH. (1995) Herniated cervical intervertebral discs spontaneously produce matrix metalloproteinases, nitric oxide, interleukin-6, and prostaglandin e2. *Spine* **20**(22): 2373–2378.

30. Montgomery DM, Brower RS. (1992) Cervical spondylotic myelopathy: Clinical syndrome and natural history. *Orthop Clin North Am* **23**(3): 487–493.

31. Goel A. (2013) Is it necessary to resect osteophytes in degenerative spondylotic myelopathy? *J Craniovertebr Junction Spine* **4**(1): 1–2.

32. Shabat S, Leitner Y, David R, Folman Y. (2012) The correlation between Spurling test and imaging studies in detecting cervical radiculopathy. *J Neuroimaging* **22**(4): 375–378.

33. Thoomes EJ, van Geest S, van der Windt DA, *et al.* (2018) Value of physical tests in diagnosing cervical radiculopathy: A systematic review. *Spine J* **18**(1): 179–189.

34. Iyer S, Kim HJ. (2016) Cervical radiculopathy. *Curr Rev Musculoskelet Med* **9**(3): 272–280.

35. Onks CA, Billy G. (2013) Evaluation and treatment of cervical radiculopathy. *Prim Care* **40**(4): 837–848, vii–viii.

36. Latka D, Miekisiak G, Jarmuzek P, *et al.* (2016) Treatment of degenerative cervical spondylosis with radiculopathy: Clinical practice guidelines endorsed by the Polish Society of Spinal Surgery. *Neurol Neurochir Pol* **50**(2): 109–113.

37. Childress MA, Becker BA. (2016) Nonoperative management of cervical radiculopathy. *Am Fam Physician* **93**(9): 746–754.

38. Ghasemi M, Masaeli A, Rezvani M, *et al.* (2013) Oral prednisolone in the treatment of cervical radiculopathy: A randomized placebo controlled trial. *J Res Med Sci* **18**(Suppl 1): S43–S46.

39. Eubanks JD. (2010) Cervical radiculopathy: Nonoperative management of neck pain and radicular symptoms. *Am Fam Physician* **81**(1): 33–40.

40. Manchikanti L, Nampiaparampil DE, Candido KD, *et al.* (2015) Do cervical epidural injections provide long-term relief in neck and upper extremity pain? A systematic review. *Pain Physician* **18**(1): 39–60.

41. Manchikanti L, Cash KA, Pampati V, *et al.* (2013) A randomized, double-blind, active control trial of fluoroscopic cervical interlaminar epidural injections in chronic pain of cervical disc herniation: Results of a 2-year follow-up. *Pain Physician* **16**(5): 465–478.

42. Rosenkranz M, Grzyska U, Niesen W, *et al.* (2004) Anterior spinal artery syndrome following periradicular cervical nerve root therapy. *J Neurol* **251**(2): 229–231.

43. Tiso RL, Cutler T, Catania JA, Whalen K. (2004) Adverse central nervous system sequelae after selective transforaminal block: The role of corticosteroids. *Spine J* **4**(4): 468–474.

44. Duehmke RM, Hollingshead J, Cornblath DR. (2006) Tramadol for neuropathic pain. *Cochrane Database Syst Rev* **3**: CD003726.

45. Mintken PE, DeRosa C, Little T, Smith B. (2008) AAOMPT clinical guidelines: A model for standardizing manipulation terminology in physical therapy practice. *J Orthop Sports Phys Ther* **38**(3): A1–A6.

46. International Federation of Orthopaedic Manipulative Physical Therapists (IFOMPT). (2016) Educational standards in orthopaedic manipulative therapy [cited 15 Nov 2019]. Available from: www.ifompt.org/site/ifompt/IFOMPT%20Standards%20Document%20definitive%202016.pdf.

47. Young IA, Pozzi F, Dunning J, *et al.* (2019) Immediate and short-term effects of thoracic spine manipulation in patients with cervical radiculopathy: A randomized controlled trial. *J Orthop Sports Phys Ther* **49**(5): 299–309.

48. Dedering A, Peolsson A, Cleland JA, *et al.* (2018) The effects of neck-specific training versus prescribed physical activity on pain and disability in patients with cervical radiculopathy: A randomized controlled trial. *Arch Phys Med Rehabil* **99**(12): 2447–2456.

49. Graham N, Gross A, Goldsmith CH, *et al.* (2008) Mechanical traction for neck pain with or without radiculopathy. *Cochrane Database Syst Rev.* **3**: CD006408.

50. Bolesta MJ, Rechtine GR 2nd, Chrin AM. (2000) Three- and four-level anterior cervical discectomy and fusion with plate fixation: A prospective study. *Spine* **25**(16): 2040–2044; Discussion 2045–2046.

51. Emery SE, Fisher JR, Bohlman HH. (1997) Three-level anterior cervical discectomy and fusion: Radiographic and clinical results. *Spine* **22**(22): 2622–2624; Discussion 2625.

52. Hilibrand AS, Robbins M. (2004) Adjacent segment degeneration and adjacent segment disease: The consequences of spinal fusion? *Spine J* **4**(6 Suppl): 190S–194S.

53. Wong JJ, Cote P, Quesnele JJ, *et al.* (2014) The course and prognostic factors of symptomatic cervical disc herniation with radiculopathy: A systematic review of the literature. *Spine J* **14**(8): 1781–1789.

54. Sleijser-Koehorst MLS, Coppieters MW, Heymans MW, *et al.* (2018) Clinical course and prognostic models for the conservative management of cervical radiculopathy: A prospective cohort study. *Eur Spine J* **27**(11): 2710–2719.

55. Cleland JA, Fritz JM, Whitman JM, Heath R. (2007) Predictors of short-term outcome in people with a clinical diagnosis of cervical radiculopathy. *Phys Ther* **87**(12): 1619–1632.

56. Faught RW, Church EW, Halpern CH, *et al.* (2016) Long-term quality of life after posterior cervical foraminotomy for radiculopathy. *Clin Neurol Neurosurg* **142**: 22–25.

2

Cervical Radiculopathy in Chinese Medicine

OVERVIEW

This chapter introduces the aetiology and pathogenesis of cervical radiculopathy from the Chinese medicine perspective. Chinese medicine therapies for this condition, including Chinese herbal medicine, acupuncture therapy and other Chinese medicine therapies are discussed.

Introduction

Cervical spondylosis or cervical radiculopathy (CR) has not been specifically defined in the history of Chinese medicine. It is commonly seen that in classical Chinese medicine literature where treatments were recorded targeting certain symptoms. The main symptoms of CR, including neck, shoulder and arm pain, may have been described in classical literature under different categories. It is possible that some descriptions of symptoms are consistent with CR; however, these symptoms in the classical books are not defined by disease names. One possible disease name referring to CR is *Xiang bi* 项痹,[1] however, this disease name has not been well-accepted. In addition, the CR-like condition may also have been mentioned under the categories of *Bi zheng* 痹证, *Jing zheng* 痉证, or *Wei zheng* 痿证 since there are certain similarity in terms of clinical symptoms.

Examples are:

- During the Spring and Autumn and Warring States period (770 BCE to 221 BCE) it was stated in the book *Lin Shu·Jing Jin* 灵枢·经筋篇 that "the Hand-*Taiyang* musculatures starts from the end of the little finger … if this is diseased, pain appears along the ulnar side of the hand, wrist, arm, elbow until the armpit, and also around the shoulder and neck" 手太阳之筋，起于小指之上 … 其病小指支肘内锐骨后廉痛，循臂阴入腋下，腋下痛，腋后廉痛，绕肩胛引颈而痛;

- The book *Yang Ke Xin De Ji* 疡科心得集·辨缺盆疽臑痛胛痛论 (1805 CE) mentioned that "the arm pain symptoms can be caused by the combination of wind, cold and dampness, or phlegm invading meridians, or unhealed injury of tendons, or *qi* stagnation and Blood stasis lingering in the meridians" 臂痛之证，或为风寒湿所搏，或痰饮流入经隧，或因挈重伤筋所致，或因气血凝滞经络不行而作痛;

- The book *Yi Shu* 医述 (1826 CE) stated that "long-term fatigue may damage *yang*, when meridians are blocked, pain occurs in shoulder and arm, it should be treated with herbs with spicy and sweet flavour, assisted with certain herbs leading the effects to relevant meridians … if patients present symptoms of pain in the elbow, arm and wrist, stiffness in the neck and difficulty in turning one's neck, and accompanied with headaches and shoulder pain that radiates to the small finger, they can be treated by stimulating the acupuncture points of SI2 *Qiangu* 前谷; if patients present symptoms of shoulder pain and difficulty in putting on/taking off clothes, and if pain in the radialis side of their arms and wrists limits their range of motion, they can be treated by stimulating the acupuncture points of SI5 *Yanggu* 阳谷" (劳倦伤阳, 脉络凝塞, 肩臂作痛者, 以辛甘为君, 佐以循经入络之品 … 臂, 腕中痛, 颈肿不可以顾, 头项急痛眩, 淫泺肩胛小指痛, 前谷主之 … 肩痛, 不可自带衣, 臂腕外侧痛不举, 阳谷主之); and

- In *Zheng Zhi Lei Cai* 类证治裁 (1839 CE), a Chinese herbal medicine (CHM) formula named *Juan bi tang* 蠲痹汤 was recorded to treat arm pain caused by dampness and *Bi* 痹 disease in the meridian (臂痛, 湿痹经络者, 蠲痹汤).

Aetiology and Pathogenesis

The understanding of CR in modern Chinese medicine is based on modern knowledge of the anatomy. It explains that the fundamental cause of CR is degenerative changes in the spine and there is a close association between the development of CR and the twelve meridian musculatures (the muscles along the regular meridians). According to modern Chinese medicine osteology and traumatology, the appearance of CR is caused by the abnormality of meridian musculatures, which is commonly caused by injuries.[2] For example, long-term inappropriate posture or acute neck injury will lead to tightness or spasms in the cervical muscles, hence the local area blood supply may decrease and the muscles, dynamic balance will be affected. Progressively, these will further affect the cervical intervertebral discs and narrow the intervertebral spaces. In addition, local ligamentous laxity will affect spinal stability and osteophyte formation (bone spurs) will slowly develop. These will further worsen the cervical intervertebral disc degeneration and the impairment of the cervical musculatures. In sum, a static and dynamic imbalance is the main cause of the occurrence and progression of CR.[3]

On the basis of the Chinese medicine meridian musculature theory, the musculatures that are related to CR are: Foot *Tai yang* musculatures 足太阳经筋, Foot *Shao yang* musculatures 足少阳经筋, Foot *Shao yin* musculatures 足少阴经筋, Hand *Tai yang* musculatures 手太阳经筋, Hand *Shao yang* musculatures 手少阳经筋, and Hand *Yang ming* musculatures 手阳明经筋.[4]

People whose jobs involve repetitive neck motions, inappropriate postures or excessive overhead work that place extra stress on their necks are likely to suffer from this condition, as well as those who have had previous neck injuries.

The commonly seen causality and aetiology of this disease are described next.[4–6]

Weak Constitution 体质虚弱

Cervical radiculopathy is very common and worsens with age. A weak constitution and ageing will cause Liver and Kidney deficiency, *qi* and Blood deficiency, weakness of bones and tendons, and insecurity of the muscular interstices; therefore, it is likely that external pathogens will invade. Long-term illness will also cause deficiency of defensive *qi* and, therefore, external pathogens, including wind, cold and heat can easily invade and linger in the cervical tendons, bones and meridians. It is worth noting that ageing is the common fundamental reason behind the aetiology and pathogenesis of CR.

Muscle Strain or Injury 劳损外伤

Chronic muscle strain or injury is usually caused by long-term inappropriate posture, which will lead to the disharmony of *qi* and Blood, and the blockage of meridians; furthermore, Blood and phlegm stasis will occur and impair the Liver, Kidney and Governing Vessel (GV) meridians. When these pathogens accumulate, the corresponding symptoms will linger and become difficult to cure.[5]

External Pathogens 外邪入侵

If a person is living or working in a cold and humid environment, the coldness and dampness may accumulate in the body over a long period of time. More specifically, if the neck and shoulder are not covered properly to keep them warm in a cold environment, the coldness and dampness may invade the muscle and meridians in these regions. This will lead to *qi* stagnation and Blood stasis in the neck/shoulders and cause pain symptoms. Such symptoms are more common in people who are aged or of a weak constitution.[6]

It should be noted that the occurrence and development of CR is a long-term course, and the causality of this disease is a combination of various factors. The fundamental cause of CR is the impairment of tendons, musculatures and bones, as well as the disharmony of *qi* and Blood. In the early stage, wind, cold and dampness that linger in musculatures and meridians will cause blockages and hence pain will appear, while in the late stage, the long-term illness will consume *qi* and Blood, and even cause *qi* deficiency and Blood stasis, hence the pain becomes chronic and difficult to eliminate.

In sum, the aetiology and pathogenesis of this condition are considered to be deficient *Ben* in combination with excess *Biao* 本虚标实. The deficient *Ben* is due to Liver, Kidney, *qi* or Blood deficiency caused by a weak constitution, ageing or chronic strain in the body, while the excess *Biao* is usually the invasion of wind-cold-dampness or accidental injury of the muscles.[4]

Chinese Medicine Syndrome Differentiation and Treatments

The Chinese medicine treatments for CR recommended by the following contemporary clinical guidelines, textbooks and experts, monographs are summarised:

- *Clinical Guideline of* Xiang Bi *(Cervical Spondylosis)* 骨伤科项痹病(神经根型颈椎病) 诊疗方案;[1]
- *Evidence-based Guidelines of Clinical Practice in Chinese Medicine* 中医循证临床实践指南 — 专科专病;[7]
- *Evidence-based Guidelines of Clinical Practice with Acupuncture and Moxibustion: Cervical Radiculopathy* 循证针灸临床实践指南: 神经根型颈椎病;[8]
- *The Standard of Chinese Medicine Diagnosis and Treatment Effect Evaluation* 中医病证诊断疗效标准;[9]
- *Tendon Traumatology in Chinese Medicine* 中医筋伤学;[10]
- *The Diagnosis and Treatment in Chinese Medicine Osteology and Traumatology* 骨伤科专病中医临床诊治;[5]
- *Advanced Textbook of Chinese Medicine Osteology and Traumatology* 中医骨伤学高级教程;[6]
- *Clinical Experience of Shi Yang-shan, the National Chinese Medicine Master* 第二届国医大师临床经验实录国医大师石仰山;[11] and
- *Li Ding-kun's Ba Duan Gong Exercise* 林定坤健体八段功.[12]

Common Chinese medicine therapies are CHM, acupuncture and other types of Chinese medicine therapies such as *tuina* 推拿 and the cupping therapy. The Chinese medicine syndrome differentiation approach should be applied for oral CHM and the acupuncture therapy.

Oral Chinese Herbal Medicine Treatment

Wind-Cold Blocking Meridians 风寒痹阻

Symptoms: Neck, shoulder and arm numbness and pain, which may radiate to the forearm; headaches with a heavy feeling; neck stiffness with a reduced range of motion; and an aversion to cold and wind. Light-red tongue body, thin white tongue coating, and a tight and wiry pulse.[1]

Treatment principle: Dispelling wind and cold 祛风散寒, and promoting Blood circulation to remove meridian obstruction 活血通络.

Formulae: Modified *Qiang huo sheng shi tang* 羌活胜湿汤,[1] *Shu feng huo xue tang* 疏风活血汤[5] or *Juan bi tang* 蠲痹汤.[7]

Herbs: *Qiang huo sheng shi tang* 羌活胜湿汤: *Qiang huo* 羌活, *du huo* 独活, *gao ben* 藁本, *fang feng* 防风, *zhi gan cao* 炙甘草, *chuan xiong* 川芎, and *man jing zi* 蔓荆子. *Shu feng huo xue tang* 疏风活血汤: *Qiang huo* 羌活, *du huo* 独活, *fang feng* 防风, *bai zhi* 白芷, *ge gen* 葛根, *sheng ma* 升麻, *hong hua* 红花, *tao ren* 桃仁, *dang gui* 当归, *chuan xiong* 川芎, *bai shao* 白芍, and *gan cao* 甘草. *Juan bi tang* 蠲痹汤: *Qiang huo* 羌活, *jiang huang* 姜黄, *dang gui* 当归, *huang qi* 黄芪, *chi shao* 赤芍, *fang feng* 防风, and *gan cao* 甘草. For severe pain, add *yuan hu* 元胡.

Analysis of herbs: The functions of herbs used in these formulae mainly are: *Qiang huo* 羌活, *du huo* 独活 and *bai shao* 白芍: Eliminate wind and dampness, and ease joint movement; *Fang feng* 防风, *bai zhi* 白芷, *gao ben* 藁本, and *man jing zi* 蔓荆子: Eliminate wind and dampness as well as reducing pain; *Ge gen* 葛根 and *sheng ma* 升麻: Eliminate external pathogens and reducing neck pain; *Hong hua* 红花, *tao ren* 桃仁, *dang gui* 当归, and *chuan xiong* 川芎: Activate *qi* and Blood movement; *Huang qi* 黄芪: Tonifies *qi*; *jiang huang* 姜黄: Removes Blood stasis, soothes meridians and relieves pain; and *gan cao* 甘草: Harmonises all herbs.

Qi Stagnation and Blood Stasis 气滞血瘀

Symptoms: Long-term, localised sharp and lingering neck, shoulder and arm pain; the pain may be severe and worsen during the night and may be accompanied by numbness and hypaesthesia. A dark-coloured tongue body and wiry pulse.[1]

Treatment principle: Promoting *qi* to activate Blood 行气活血, removing meridian obstruction and relieving pain 通络止痛.

Formulae: Modified *Tao hong si wu tang* 桃红四物汤加减[1] or *Shen tong zhu yu tang* 身痛逐瘀汤.[5]

Herbs: *Tao hong si wu tang* 桃红四物汤: *Shu di huang* 熟地黄, *dang gui* 当归, *bai shao* 白芍, *chuan xiong* 川芎, *tao ren* 桃仁, and *hong hua* 红花. *Sheng tong zhu yu tang* 身痛逐瘀汤: *Tao ren* 桃仁, *hong hua* 红花, *dang gui* 当归, *wu ling zhi* 五灵脂, *di long* 地龙, *chuan xiong* 川芎, *xiang fu* 香附, *qiang huo* 羌活, *qin jiao* 秦艽, *niu xi* 牛膝, *mo yao* 没药 and *gan cao* 甘草.

Analysis of herbs: The functions of herbs used in these formulae mainly are: *Tao ren* 桃仁, *hong hua* 红花, *dang gui* 当归 and *chuan xiong* 川芎: Activate Blood movement to remove Blood stasis; *Shu di huang* 熟地黄 and *shao yao* 芍药: Tonify *yin* and Blood; *Qin jiao* 秦艽 and *qiang huo* 羌活: Eliminate wind and dampness; *Mo yao* 没药, *wu ling zhi* 五灵脂 and *xiang fu* 香附: Promote *qi* and Blood movement as well as relieving pain; *Niu xi* 牛膝 and *di long* 地龙: Soothe meridians and joints; and *gan cao* 甘草: Harmonises all herbs.

Phlegm and Dampness Blocking Meridians 痰湿阻络

Symptoms: Dizziness with blurred vision, heaviness in the head, numbness of limbs and a decreased appetite. A dark-red tongue body that is thick with a greasy coating, and a wiry and slippery pulse.[1]

Treatment principle: Clearing dampness and removing phlegm 祛湿化痰, removing meridian obstruction and relieving pain 通络止痛.

Formulae: Modified *Ban xia bai zhu tian ma tang* 半夏白术天麻汤.[1]

Herbs: *Ban xia* 半夏 *bai zhu* 白术, *tian ma* 天麻, *fu ling* 茯苓, *ju hong* 橘红, *bai zhu* 白术, *gan cao* 甘草, etc.

Analysis of herbs: *Tian ma* 天麻: Calms the Liver, eliminates wind and relieves dizziness; *bai zhu* 白术 and *fu ling* 茯苓: Strengthen the Spleen and clear dampness; *ju hong* 橘红: Regulates *qi* and eliminates phlegm; and *gan cao* 甘草: Harmonises all herbs.

Liver and Kidney Deficiency 肝肾不足

Symptoms: Pain and numbness in the shoulder and neck region, tight limbs, an unsteady walk accompanied by dizziness, tinnitus, a dry mouth, macritus, a red face, irritability, poor sleep, a bitter mouth and dry throat, dry stool and little urine. A red and dry tongue, and a wiry and thin pulse.[1]

Treatment principle: Tonifying Liver and Kidney 补益肝肾, and removing meridian obstruction and relieving pain 通络止痛.

Formulae: Modified *Shen qi wan* 肾气丸[1] or *Du huo ji sheng tang* 独活寄生汤.[7]

Herbs: *Shen qi wan* 肾气丸: *Shu di huang* 熟地黄, *shan yao* 山药, *shan zhu yu* 山茱萸, *mu dan pi* 牡丹皮, *fu ling* 茯苓, *ze xie* 泽泻, *gui zhi* 桂枝 and *fu zi* 附子. *Du huo ji sheng tang* 独活寄生汤: *Du huo* 独活, *sang ji sheng* 桑寄生, *du Zhong* 杜仲, *niu xi* 牛膝, *xi xin* 细辛, *qin jiao* 秦艽, *fu ling* 茯苓, *rou gui* 肉桂, *fang feng* 防风, *chuan xiong* 川芎, *ren sheng* 人参, *gan cao* 甘草, *dang gui* 当归, *bai shao* 白芍 and *shu di huang* 熟地黄. For severe pain, consider adding *di long* 地龙, *tao ren* 桃仁 and *hong hua* 红花; for severe cold pathogen invasion, add *fu zi* 附子; for severe dampness accumulation, add *fang ji* 防己.

Analysis of herbs: *Fu zi* 附子, *gui zhi* 桂枝, *ren shen* 人参 and *rou gui* 肉桂: Tonify *yang*; *Di huang* 地黄, *shan zhu yu* 山茱萸 and *shan yao* 山药: Tonify Kidney, Liver and Spleen *yin*; *Ze xie* 泽泻 and *fu ling* 茯苓: Clear dampness and promote diuresis; *Du huo* 独活 and *xi xin* 细辛: Tonify and soothe Kidney meridian; *Qin jiao* 秦艽 and *fang feng* 防风: Eliminate wind and soothe meridians; *Sang ji sheng*

桑寄生: Eliminates wind and clears dampness; *Du zhu* 杜仲 and *niu xi* 牛膝: Tonify and strengthen bones and tendons; *Chuan xiong* 川芎, *dang gui* 当归, *bai shao* 白芍 and *dan pi* 丹皮: Tonify Blood, activate Blood movement and reduce Blood stasis; and *gan cao* 甘草: Harmonises all herbs.

Qi and Blood Deficiency 气血亏虚

Symptoms: Long-term lingering disease with dull pain or numbness and hypaesthesia, tiredness and weakness; symptoms may get worse after physical work. Accompanied by dizziness, blurred version and pale complexion. A pale tongue body with little coating, and a thin and weak pulse.[1]

Treatment principle: Tonifying *qi* and warming meridians 益气温经, and harmonising Blood and relieving *Bi* symptoms 和血通痹.

Formulae: Modified *Huang qi gui zhi wu wu tang* 黄芪桂枝五物汤[5] and *Ba zhen tang* 八珍汤.[7]

Herbs: *Huang qi gui zhi wu wu tang* 黄芪桂枝五物汤: *Huang qi* 黄芪, *shao yao* 芍药, *gui zhi* 桂枝, *sheng jiang* 生姜, *da zao* 大枣, etc., *Ba zhen tang* 八珍汤: *Bai zhu* 白术, *fu ling* 茯苓, *ren shen* 人参, *gan cao* 甘草, *dang gui* 当归, *chuan xiong* 川芎, *shu di huang* 熟地黄 and *bai shao* 白芍. For severe pain, consider adding *di long* 地龙, *tao ren* 桃仁 and *hong hua* 红花.

Analysis of herbs: *Huang qi* 黄芪 and *gui zhi* 桂枝: Tonify *qi* and *yang*; *Sheng jiang* 生姜 and *da zao* 大枣: Tonify Spleen and Blood; *Ren shen* 人参 and *shu di huang* 熟地黄: Tonify *qi* and Blood; *Bai zhu* 白术 and *fu ling* 茯苓: Tonify Spleen and clear dampness; *Dang gui* 当归, *bai shao* 白芍 and *chuan xiong* 川芎: Tonify Blood and activate Blood movement; and *gan cao* 甘草: Harmonises all herbs.

Topical Chinese Herbal Medicine Treatment

Topical CHM can be applied on a localised area via a few different approaches. The common approaches are topical ointments, externally used plasters, externally applied herbal liquids, CHM bathing or steaming, CHM iontophoresis, and CHM heat packs.[1]

Shu jin huo luo yao gao 舒筋活络药膏, *Huo xue gao* 活血膏, *Wen jing tong luo gao* 温经通络膏, *Gou pi gao* 狗皮膏, etc., are commonly used CHM sticking plasters that can be applied directly onto the skin. These can be used on the neck and shoulder areas once a day, and be removed or replaced according to skin reactions and symptoms. It is suggested that if there is any reaction indicating an occurrence of contact dermatitis, the plasters should be removed immediately.[10]

Topical CHM can also be applied as creams, ointments, tincture preparations, etc. Commonly used liquid CHM preparations that contain alcohol are *Huo xue jiu* 活血酒 and *Zheng gu shui* 正骨水, while oiling agents such as *Die da wan hua you* 跌打万花油, *Zheng hong hua you* 正红花油, *Huo luo you* ointment 活络油膏, *Suan tong you* 酸痛油, etc., are also commonly used since they are easy to apply and cause minimum skin irritation. These topical CHM preparations can be applied before or after *tuina* 推拿 therapy.[10]

CHM formulae such as *Hai tong pi tang* 海桐皮汤 and *Shang zhi sun shang xi fang* 上肢损伤洗方 are recommended as a bathing or steaming therapy. These CHM formulae are made as decoctions: A steaming therapy is first applied when using the decoction while it is hot, then the bathing therapy is applied when the decoction cools down. Patients can apply the decoction on localised areas once or twice a day for 15–30 minutes each time. Caution should be taken to avoid skin scalding.[10]

The topical CHM formula *Kan li sha* 坎离砂, single herb *wu zhu yu* 吴茱萸 or coarse salt can be used externally as heat packs on the cervical region.[10]

CHM iontophoresis is a modern form of topical CHM administration. Using an iontophoresis apparatus, a decoction or liquid form of CHM is applied externally through pairs of electrodes. *Dang gui zhu she ye* 当归注射液, *Dan shen zhu she ye* 丹参注射液 or decoctions of other commonly used CHM formulae can be selected for this method. Firstly, wet some pads with the CHM liquid and attach them to the electrodes, then place these electrodes on the skin and turn on the ion-conduction machine at an intensity below the patient's tolerance threshold. Two points (one pair of electrodes) can be used in each session for 30 minutes daily, for five days; the following two days are spent resting. One to two rounds are usually needed. Cervical EX-B2 *Jiaji* points 颈夹脊穴, GB20 *Fengchi* 风池, GB21 *Jianjing* 肩井, GV14 *Dazhui* 大椎 and SI11 *Tianzong* 天宗 are commonly used in clinical practice for the management of CR.[13]

Acupuncture Therapies

Acupuncture therapies used to treat CR include acupuncture needling, moxibustion and other acupuncture-related therapies. In current Chinese medicine clinical practice, there are multiple styles of acupuncture needling, such as traditional body acupuncture and modern styles, including abdominal acupuncture, scalp acupuncture, etc. Moxibustion can be applied as sticks or cones, as well as via some modern moxibustion devices. In addition, ear acupuncture or acupressure, a form of acupuncture therapy based on reflexology theory, can also be used as a treatment for CR.[8]

The benefit of acupuncture therapy for treating CR is that it may reduce pain and relieve the symptoms of numbness quickly. In the acute stage of CR, the principle of acupuncture treatment is expelling wind and cold pathogens, activating Blood and reducing pain; in the chronic stage of CR, the treatment principle is to unblock meridians, eliminate stagnation and reduce pain; while in the recovery stage of CR, treatment should focus on tonifying *qi* and the Blood, Kidney and Liver.[8]

Body Acupuncture

The principle of acupuncture point selection is: the points on a localised area (neck and shoulder region) serve as the main points used in the treatment of CR. These include cervical EX-B2 *Jiaji* points 颈夹脊穴 (according to the affected cervical segment) and local *Ashi* points 阿是穴, which remove *qi* stagnation and Blood stasis and reduce pain. In addition, distal points that have the function of reducing symptoms of pain, numbness, weakness and muscle atrophy should be used according to patients, complaints.[8]

Main points: Cervical EX-B2 *Jiaji* points 颈夹脊穴 according to the affected cervical segment, local *Ashi* points 阿是穴, GV14 *Dazhui* 大椎, BL10 *Tianzhu* 天柱, SI3 *Houxi* 后溪 and EX-HN15 *Jing bailao* 颈百劳.[8]

Additional points according to symptoms:

- Shoulder soreness, add BL11 *Dazhu* 大杼 and SI11 *Tianzong* 天宗;
- Numbness on the radial side of the forearm, add LI11 *Quchi* 曲池, LI4 *Hegu* 合谷, LI2 *Erjian* 二间 and LI3 *Sanjian* 三间;
- Numbness on the middle part of the forearm, add LU5 *Chize* 尺泽, TE4 *Yangchi* 阳池 and TE1 *Guanchong* 关冲; and
- Numbness on the medial side of the forearm, add SI8 *Xiaohai* 小海 and TE3 *Zhongzhu* 中渚.

Additional points according to Chinese medicine syndrome differentiation:

- Wind-cold blocking meridians, add BL12 *Fengmen* 风门 and GV16 *Fengfu* 风府; and
- *Qi* stagnation and Blood stasis, add BL17 *Geshu* 膈俞, LI4 *Hegu* 合谷 and LR3 *Taichong* 太冲.

Method: Needling of cervical EX-B2 *Jiaji* points 颈夹脊穴 should direct the needle sensation to the neck and shoulder region; for GV14 *Dazhui* 大椎 and EX-HN15 *Jing baibao* 颈百劳, at a perpendicular angle of 1–1.5 *cun*, direct the needle sensation to the shoulder and arm; apply a regular acupuncture technique on other points. During the needle-retaining time, a *Teding Diancibo Pu* (TDP) lamp can be applied to warm up the neck region.

Treatment duration: Once daily, six sessions as one course, usually three to five courses are required.[8]

Electroacupuncture

Point selection follows the same principle as stated above.

Method: Once the *deqi* 得气 sensation is achieved, select two to three pairs of sensitive points for electroacupuncture for 30 minutes.[8]

Treatment duration: Once daily, six sessions as one course, usually requires three to five courses.[8]

Heat-Sensitive Moxibustion

Points: Select sensitive points on the neck and shoulder region.

Method: Apply moxibustion on the sensitive points using moxibustion sticks for 10 to 20 minutes in one session.

Treatment duration: Once daily, 10 sessions as one course. This method can be applied for multiple courses until the symptoms are relieved.[8]

Ear Acupressure

Points: AH12 *Jing* 颈, AH13 *Jingzhui* 颈椎, TF4 *Shenmen* 神门, AT4 *Pizhixia* 皮质下, CO10 *Shen* 肾, EX-HN6 *Erjian* 耳尖, SF4, 5 *Jian* 肩, SF3 *Zhou* 肘, SF2 *Wan* 腕 and SF1 *Zhi* 指.

Method: The use of adhesive tape to place ear pellets on up to two to five relevant points each time. Patients are told to press the pellets three to four times a day for a minute per point or until one reaches an unbearable level of pain.[8]

Treatment duration: Three times a week, 10 sessions as one course. This method can be applied for multiple courses until the symptoms are relieved.[8]

Other Chinese Medicine Therapies

Some other Chinese medicine therapies applied externally are commonly used for the prevention and treatment of CR.

Cupping

Cupping therapy can be applied on the shoulder/neck area, such as on the points GB21 *Jianjing* 肩井, GV14 *Dazhui* 大椎 or *Ashi* points

阿是穴. Cups can be applied after acupuncture treatment and be retained for 15–20 minutes.[14]

Tuina 推拿 *Therapy*

There are two types of Chinese medicine *tuina* 推拿 therapy: (1) Relaxing manipulation therapy, and (2) Spinal adjusting manipulating therapy.[1]

Relaxing manipulating therapy

As recommended by the Chinese medicine clinical guideline,[1] there are three types of manipulation methods that can be used to relax local tissues and muscles:

- One-finger Zen massage method 一指禅, hand rolling, pushing, tapping, etc.: One or more of these common massage methods can be used to relax the local muscles, with or without adjusting manipulating therapy in combination;
- Adjusting the GV meridian 通调督脉法: The practitioner can use his thumb to press certain acupuncture points of the GV meridian such as GV16 *Fengfu* 风府, followed by GV14 *Dazhui* 大椎, GV 9 *Zhiyang* 至阳 and GV4 *Mingmen* 命门. Then he can perform a kneading massage on the EX-B2 *Jiaji* points 夹脊穴 of the T1 to T12 level, followed by another kneading massage on the Bladder meridian. These actions should be repeated three times. The intensity of the massage should be controlled within the level of the patient getting sensations of warmness, soreness and distention, or of sensations that radiate along the meridians; and
- Intermittent manual traction: With the patient lying in a supine position, the physician puts one hand on the patient's occiput and holds the patient's chin with the other. He then pulls the patient's head for 2 to 3 minutes, before relaxing for 5 to 10 seconds. This manual traction procedure can be repeated three to five times.

Spinal adjusting manipulation therapy

There are various *tuina* 推拿 therapies used in clinical practice in the treatment of CR. They were developed from therapies recorded in classical literature, such as the Qing dynasty imperial palace "bone-setting therapy" 清宫正骨疗法, Dr. Shi's "bone-setting therapy" (orthopaedic manipulation therapy) and Dr. Wei's *tuina* 推拿 therapy. In this chapter, a few commonly used therapies are introduced: Rotation-traction manipulation,[15] rotation-pulling-pushing manipulation in the sitting position,[16] rotation manipulation,[1] and Dr. Shi's "bone-setting therapy".[11]

- Rotation-traction manipulation[15]

The patient remains in an upright sitting position and relaxes his muscles. First, the physician performs some gentle *tuina* 推拿 techniques to relax the local muscles, which include pressing, kneading and rolling methods for 5 to 10 minutes. Secondly, under the physician's instruction, the patient slowly turns his head to one side to its physiological limit and then lowers his head to move his chin to be as close to the chest as possible. The physician then uses his arm to hold the patient's head with the chelidon and while supporting the patient,s chin firmly, pulls the patient's head up gently and keeps pulling for three to five seconds. Then the physician performs a quick and strong upward pull. This quick pulling may induce a cracking sound, which indicates a successful manipulation. Thereafter, the physician loosens his forearm gradually and performs the gentle relaxing manipulation therapy again. This therapy can be applied once in two days with each session requiring 10 to 15 minutes in total.

- Rotation-pulling-pushing Manipulation in Sitting Position[16]

Using the C6 spinous process tilting right as an example, the patient first sits upright, and the physician stands behind the patient. The physician then locates his right thumb on the left side of the patient's C6 spinous process while holding the patient's chin firmly with his left hand. The patient needs to lower his head slightly (of up to 15° of a head's flexion). The physician then pushes the patient's head against his chest and turns the patient's head 45° to the left, with his right thumb quickly pushing the C6 spinous process towards the left simultaneously; at this moment a cracking sound can be heard. When all these manipulations are completed, the physician slowly moves the patient's head and neck back to the normal position.

• Rotation manipulation[1]

If the CR occurs in the upper cervical segments, the physician asks the patient to lower his head to 15° of flexion while in a sitting position, and then turn his head to the left or right of its physiological limit (approximately 80°). Then, the physician rotates the patient's head quickly and accurately in the same direction; a cracking sound can be heard, indicating a successful manipulation. If the CR occurs in the middle cervical segments, the physician performs this method with the patient keeping his head in a neutral position. If the CR occurs in the lower cervical segments, this method should be performed when the patient lowers his head to 30–45° of flexion.

• Dr. Shi's bone-setting therapy[11]

The classical terminology of "bone-setting therapy" 正骨疗法 refers to the orthopaedic manipulation therapy. The method for Dr. Shi's bone-setting therapy is: The patient sits upright and the physician stands behind the patient and examines the patient's neck carefully. In the situation where the patient's neck slightly bends laterally (e.g., bending towards the right side), the physician places his left hand on the patient's left shoulder with his right hand on top of the patient's head. The physician pushes the patient's head towards the right to its physiological limit and then performs a quick and powerful push; a cracking sound may occur. After this, the physician moves the patient's head to an upright position, holds it with one arm, and with the chelidon supporting the patient's chin firmly, places the opposite hand on the patient's occiput and performs a quick and strong upward pull. At the end, the physician uses both hands to quickly pull the patient's head up, with his thumbs pressing the acupuncture point GB20 *Fengchi* 风池 and palms holding the patient's cheeks.

Daoyi 导引 *Exercise*

The *daoyi* 导引 exercise refers to a series of body and mind unity exercises. It can be interpreted as a combination of gentle physical exercise and *qigong* therapy.[12] A few different types of *daoyi* 导引 therapies are recommended to be beneficial for the prevention and treatment of CR, such as the *Ba duan jin* 八段锦 exercise, Shi's twelve-word *Qigong* therapy 施氏十二字养生功[17] and Lin Ding-kun,s *Ba duan qigong* therapy 林定坤健体八段功.[12] In particular, the *Ba duan jin* 八段锦 exercise and one particular exercise of Lin Ding-kun's *Ba duan qigong* therapy, namely 双手托天理三焦 (both hands pushing up to regulate the three-*Jiao*), are considered effective for the prevention and treatment of CR.

Prevention and Lifestyle Adjustment

Lifestyle Adjustment

Avoiding inappropriate sitting or sleeping postures, overexertion and wind-cold invasion, particularly on the neck and shoulder regions, may prevent the development of CR.[10]

Appropriate Postures During the Day

While sitting, keep the upper body straight, avoid sitting with a hunch and keep one's computer screen or book at eye level. Avoid reading or staring at a computer screen for a long time; it is suggested to change one's posture every 30–45 minutes and perform a gentle movement exercise of the neck.[12] While walking or standing, keep the upper body straight and head facing forward.

Sleeping Posture

Selecting a suitable pillow before going to sleep is essential for patients with CR. The pillow should be of the same height as the shoulder when lying on one's side; the head should be slightly raised when lying on the back. Avoid reading when lying in bed.[12]

Psychological Management

Cervical radiculopathy is a recurrent condition. Severe pain may affect patients, quality of life and generate irritability. Explaining the mechanisms and management thoroughly and guiding patients to perform regular exercises may help them to remain confident and reduce irritability, therefore improving their quality of life.[10]

Tables 2.1, 2.2 and 2.3 are summaries of oral CHM formulae, topical CHM formulae, and acupuncture and other Chinese medicine therapies for the treatment of CR.

Table 2.1. Summary of Oral Chinese Herbal Medicine Formulae for Cervical Radiculopathy

Syndrome Differentiation	Treatment Principle	Chinese Herbal Medicine Formulae
Wind-cold blocking meridians 风寒痹阻	Dispelling wind and cold 祛风散寒 and promoting Blood circulation to remove meridian obstruction 活血通络	Modified *Qiang huo sheng shi tang* 羌活胜湿汤, *Shu feng huo xue tang* 疏风活血汤 or *Juan bi tang* 蠲痹汤
Qi stagnation and Blood stasis 气滞血瘀	Promoting *qi* to activate Blood 行气活血, and removing meridian obstruction and relieving pain 通络止痛	Modified *Tao hong si wu tang* 桃红四物汤加减 or *Shen tong zhu yu tang* 身痛逐瘀汤
Phlegm and dampness blocking meridians 痰湿阻络	Clearing dampness and removing phlegm 祛湿化痰, and removing meridian obstruction and relieving pain 通络止痛	Modified *Ban xia bai zhu tian ma tang* 半夏白术天麻汤
Liver and Kidney deficiency 肝肾不足	Tonifying Liver and Kidney 补益肝肾, and removing meridian obstruction and relieving pain 通络止痛	Modified *Shen qi wan* 肾气丸 or *Du huo ji sheng tang* 独活寄生汤
Qi and Blood deficiency 气血亏虚	Tonifying *qi* and warming meridians 益气温经, and harmonising Blood and relieving *Bi* symptoms 和血通痹	Modified *Huang qi gui zhi wu wu tang* 黄芪桂枝五物汤 or *Ba zhen tang* 八珍汤

Table 2.2. Summary of Topical Chinese Herbal Medicine Formulae for Cervical Radiculopathy

Topical Application Method	CHM Formula
CHM sticking plaster	*Shu jin huo luo yao gao* 舒筋活络药膏, *Huo xue gao* 活血膏, *Wen jing tong luo gao* 温经通络膏 and *Gou pi gao* 狗皮膏
Topical application before or after *tuina* 推拿 therapy	*Huo xue jiu* 活血酒, *Zheng gu shui* 正骨水, while oiling agents such as *Die da wan hua you* 跌打万花油, *Zheng hong hua you* 正红花油, *Huo luo you gao* 活络油膏 and *Suan tong you* 酸痛油
CHM bathing or steaming therapy	*Hai tong pi tang* 海桐皮汤 and *Shang zhi sun shang xi fang* 上肢损伤洗方
CHM heat pack	CHM formula *Kan li sha* 坎离砂 and single herb *wu zhu yu* 吴茱萸 or coarse salt
CHM iontophoresis	*Dang gui zhu she ye* 当归注射液, *Dan shen zhu she ye* 丹参注射液 or other CHM formula decoctions

CHM: Chinese herbal medicine.

Table 2.3. Summary of Acupuncture and Other Chinese Medicine Therapies for Cervical Radiculopathy

Type of Therapy	Details
Regular acupuncture	Main points: Cervical EX-B2 *Jiaji* points 颈夹脊穴 according to the affected cervical segment, local *Ashi* points 阿是穴, GV14 *Dazhui* 大椎, BL10 *Tianzhu* 天柱, SI3 *Houxi* 后溪 and EX-HN15 *Jing bailao* 颈百劳.
Electroacupuncture	As above.
Heat-sensitive moxibustion	Select sensitive points on the neck and shoulder region.
Ear acupressure	AH12 *Jing* 颈, AH13 *Jingzhui* 颈椎, TF4 *Shenmen* 神门, AT4 *Pizhixia* 皮质下, CO10 *Shen* 肾, EX-HN6 *Erjian* 耳尖, SF4,5 *Jian* 肩, SF3 *Zhou* 肘, SF2 *Wan* 腕 and SF1 *Zhi* 指.
Cupping	On the shoulder/neck area, points of GB21 *Jianjing* 肩井, GV14 *Dazhui* 大椎 or *Ashi* points 阿是穴.

(Continued)

Table 2.3. (*Continued*)

Type of Therapy	Details
Tuina 推拿 therapy (relaxing manipulating therapy)	Common massage methods, adjusting GV meridian 通调督脉法 and intermittent manual traction.
Tuina 推拿 therapy (spinal adjusting manipulation therapy)	Rotation-traction manipulation, rotation-pulling-pushing manipulation in sitting position, rotation manipulation, and Shi's bone-setting therapy.
Daoyi 导引 exercise	*Ba duan jin* 八段锦 exercise, Shi's twelve words *qigong* therapy 施氏十二字养生功 and Lin Ding-kun's *Ba duan qigong* therapy 林定坤健体八段功.

References

1. 国家中医药管理局. (2017) 国家中医药管理局办公室关于印发中风病 (脑梗死) 等92个病种中医临床路径和中医诊疗方案的通知: 骨伤科项痹病 (神经根型颈椎病) 中医诊疗方案. Available from: http://yzs.satcm. gov.cn/gongzuodongtai/2018-03-24/2651.html.

2. 方维, 赵勇. (2017) 颈椎病发病与软组织张力的相关性探讨. *中国中医基础医学杂志* **23**(01): 100–102.

3. 王拥军. (1997) 施杞教授关于颈椎病理论与临床的探讨. *中国中医骨伤科* (03): 62–64.

4. 孟凡萍, 胡志俊, 钱雪华, *et al.* (2011) 从经筋气血理论指导针刀治疗神经根型颈椎病的认识. *辽宁中医杂志* **38**(07): 1425–1427.

5. 林定坤, 杨海韵, 刘金文主编. (2013) 骨伤科专病中医临床诊治 (3rd edn.). 人民卫生出版社, 北京.

6. 孙树椿主编. (2018) 中医骨伤学高级教程. 中华医学电子音像出版社, 北京.

7. 中国中医科学院. (2011) 中医循证临床实践指南: 专科专病. 中国中医药出版社, 北京.

8. 中国针灸学会. (2015) 中国针灸学会标准 — 循证针灸临床实践指南: 神经根型颈椎病. 中国中医药出版社出版, 北京.

9. 国家中医药管理局. (1994) 中医病证诊断疗效标准. 南京大学出版社, 南京.

10. 黄桂成. (2016) 中医筋伤学. 中国中医药出版社, 北京.

11. 邱德华, 蔡奇文主编. (2015) 第二届国医大师临床经验实录 — 国医大师石仰山. 中国医药科技出版社, 北京.

12. 林定坤主编. (2016) 林定坤健体八段功. 广东教育出版社, 广州.

13. 刘浪琪. (2008) 中药离子导入法治疗神经根型颈椎病临床研究 (Thesis). 广州中医药大学.
14. 管恩福, 刘彦璐, 李绍旦, *et al*. (2014) 正骨手法结合刺血拔罐治疗神经根型颈椎病临床观察. *中国中医急症* **24**(08): 1418–1420.
15. 朱立国, 韩涛, 于杰, *et al*. (2018) 中医骨伤科旋提手法规范化操作传承模式初探. *中医杂志* **59**(11): 927–931.
16. 韦贵康, 韦坚, 韦理. (2009) 颈椎病整合手法具体应用及力学原理分析. *中国骨伤* **22**(09): 683–684.
17. 施杞, 吴瞍. (2000) 施杞谈颈椎病. 上海科技教育出版社, 上海.

3

Classical Chinese Medicine Literature

OVERVIEW

Classical Chinese medicine literature has provided abundant experience of the prevention and management of various health conditions and diseases. This chapter systematically summarises and evaluates the evidence obtained from classical Chinese medicine literature for cervical radiculopathy in the *Zhong Hua Yi Dian* (中华医典), one of the most comprehensive digital collections of Chinese medicine books accessible. A total of 684 citations describing treatments for cervical radiculopathy are identified. As an important component of the "whole evidence" approach, the aetiology, pathogenesis and treatments with Chinese herbal medicine, acupuncture and other Chinese medicine therapies for cervical radiculopathy are analysed and summarised.

Introduction

The earliest written records of Chinese medicine history date back to the periods of Spring and Autumn (770–476 BCE) and the Warring States (474–221 BCE). Texts from these periods describe concepts such as *yin* and *yang*, as well as giving descriptions of herbal decoctions, acupuncture and moxibustion as ways to treat health complaints.[1] Some of the experiences from classical literature contribute to the contemporary understanding and management of cervical radiculopathy (CR).

In classical Chinese medicine literature, CR was not considered a specific disease, but it may have been described under the umbrella of the *Bi* (1) disease 痹证 (impediment diseases or arthralgia). It should be pointed out that two Chinese characters pronounced *bi* the same way but have different meanings. In this chapter, these two words are denoted as *Bi* (1) 痹 (referring to a disease in Chinese medicine) and *bi* (2) 臂 (referring to the arm).

Ancient Chinese medicine practitioners started documenting manifestations possibly related to CR in the book *Huang Di Nei Jing* 黄帝内经 (474–221 BCE). In the *Su Wen·Bi Lun* 素问·痹论 section, the authors pointed out that wind, cold and dampness were the three main pathological factors generating *Bi* (1) disease 痹证.[2] In addition, symptoms possibly related to CR were also described under various terms such as *bi* (2) *tong* 臂痛 (arm pain) and *jian tong* 肩痛 (shoulder pain) in past eras. Considering that CR has been mentioned under different diseases or symptom terms, and vice versa, these diseases or symptom terms were not limited to CR, hence it is important to comprehensively search all relevant terms to identify citations referring to this condition and systematically analyse relevant treatments recorded in classical literature. A comprehensive electronic search of the *Zhong Hua Yi Dian* (ZHYD) 中华医典 "Encyclopedia of Traditional Chinese Medicine" was conducted.[3] This digitalised collection of more than 1,100 medical books is the largest currently available and is representative of other large collections of classical and pre-modern Chinese medical literature.[4]

Search Terms

In classical Chinese medicine literature, there was no specific term for CR. However, the key clinical manifestation of CR such as arm pain (*bi* (2) *tong* 臂痛), shoulder pain (*jian tong* 肩痛), elbow pain radiating to the shoulder (*zhou tong yin jian* 肘痛引肩) and radial arm and hand pain (*bi* (2) *wan wai ce tong* 臂腕外侧痛) were commonly mentioned in the vast classical literature under a number of terms. These descriptions can be obtained from the sections "*Zhu Bi* (1) *Men* 诸痹门" (impediment diseases or arthralgia), "*Zhu Tong Men* 诸痛门" (pain diseases), "*Tan Yin Men* 痰饮门" (phlegm diseases),

"*Tong Feng Men* 痛风门" (pain and wind diseases), and "*Bi* (2) *Tong* 臂痛*" (arm pain) in classical literature.

In order to identify possible examples of CR in the classical literature, contemporary Chinese medicine textbooks[2,5,6] and relevant theses[7–16] were accessed and reviewed for the search terms. A list of 37 search terms was developed after reviews by Chinese medicine specialists and experts:

- Body location terms related to CR such as *jing xiang* 颈项 (neck), *bi* (2) 臂 (arm), *shang zhi* 上肢 (upper limbs), and *bo jing* 脖颈 (neck);
- Symptom terms related to CR such as *xiang tong* 项痛 (nape pain), *bi* (2) *tong* 臂痛 (arm pain), *xiang jiang* 项强 (stiffness of the neck), *jian bei tong* 肩背痛 (shoulder and back pain), *zhi jie tong* 肢节痛 (limb pain), *jian tong* 肩痛 (shoulder pain), *jing xiang tong* 颈项痛 (neck and nape pain), *shou tong* 手痛 (hand pain), *xiang jin ji* 项筋急 (contracture of nape tendon), *bi* (2) *teng* 臂疼 (arm pain), *xiang bei tong* 项背痛 (nape and back pain), *jing jin ji* 颈筋急 (contracture of neck tendon), *ji bei tong* 脊背痛 (back pain along the spine), *jian bi* (2) *tong* 肩臂痛 (shoulder and arm pain), *shou teng tong* 手疼痛 (hand pain), *xiang bi* (2) *tong* 项臂痛 (nape and arm pain), *jia ji tong* 夹脊痛 (back pain along the spine), *jing jian tong* 颈肩痛 (neck and shoulder pain) and *shou ma* 手麻 (hand numbness); and
- General disease names related to CR such as *jing bi* (1) 颈痹 (neck impediment disease or arthralgia), *jian men* 肩门 (shoulder diseases) and *bi* (2) *zheng* 臂症 (arm disease).

Considering that general terms such as: *Bi* (1) 痹 (impediment disease or arthralgia), *tou tong* 头痛 (headache), *gu tong* 骨痛 (bone pain), *xuan yun* 眩晕 (vertigo) and *tan zheng* 痰证 (syndrome of phlegm) may refer to a broad range of diseases, eight combinations of the search terms and body location terms were included to reduce the search range. Table 3.1 presents the full list of search terms or combinations we used for the search of ZHYD.

Table 3.1. Terms Used to Identify Classical Literature Citations

Search Terms for CR in *Pinyin*	Search Terms for CR in Chinese	English Translation
Bi (1) and *xiang**	痹, 项*	Impediment disease and nape
Tou tong and *bi* (2)*	头痛, 臂*	Headache and arm
Bi (1) and *jian**	痹, 肩*	Impediment disease and shoulder
Bi (1) and *bi* (2)*	痹, 臂*	Impediment disease and arm
Gu tong and *bi* (2)*	骨痛, 臂*	Bone pain and arm
Xiang tong	项痛	Nape pain
Bi (2) *tong*	臂痛	Arm pain
Xiang jiang	项强	Stiffness of the neck
Jing xiang	颈项	Neck
Bi (2)	臂	Arm
Jian bei tong	肩背痛	Shoulder and back pain
Gu bi (1) and *bi* (2)*	骨痹, 臂*	Bone impediment disease and arm
Zhi jie tong	肢节痛	Limb pain
Xuan yun and *bi* (2) *tong**	眩晕, 臂痛*	Vertigo and arm pain
Jian tong	肩痛	Shoulder pain
Shou ma	手麻	Hand numbness
Bi jue	臂厥	Reversal of the arm
Shang zhi	上肢	Upper limbs
Jing xiang tong	颈项痛	Neck pain
Tan zheng and *bi* (2)*	痰症, 臂*	Syndrome of phlegm and arm
Shou tong	手痛	Hand pain
Xiang jin ji	项筋急	Contracture of nape tendon
Bi (2) *teng*	臂疼	Arm pain
Xiang bei tong	项背痛	Nape and back pain
Jing jin ji	颈筋急	Contracture of neck tendon
Ji bei tong	脊背痛	Back pain along the spine
Jian bi (2) *tong*	肩臂痛	Shoulder and arm pain
Shou teng tong	手疼痛	Hand pain
Bi bing	臂病	Arm disease
Jing bi (1)	颈痹	Neck impediment disease

Table 3.1.   (*Continued*)

Search Terms for CR in *Pinyin*	Search Terms for CR in Chinese	English Translation
Jian men	肩门	Shoulder diseases
Xiang bi tong	项臂痛	Nape and arm pain
Bi (2) *zheng*	臂症	Arm disease
Jia ji tong	夹脊痛	Back pain along the spine
Xiang bi (2)	项痹	Nape impediment disease
Bo jing	脖颈	Neck
Jing jian tong	颈肩痛	Neck and shoulder pain

Abbreviation: CR, cervical radiculopathy.

*Two terms were searched as a combination; two Chinese characters (痹 and 臂) are both pronounced "*bi*" but have different meanings. These are marked *bi* (1) and *bi* (2).

Procedures for Search

Search terms were entered into both the heading and text search fields of the ZHYD, and the search results were downloaded into spreadsheets. Duplicate citations, which meant that the same citation was found by multiple search terms, were excluded. A "citation" was defined as a distinct passage of text referring to one or more of the search terms. Codes were allocated for the type of citation, book and the dynasty in which they were written according to the procedures described in May *et al.*[3] Books published after 1949 (the end of the Minguo/Republic of China) were excluded. The process for searching, sorting and analysing information from the classical literature is illustrated in Fig. 3.1.

Data Coding and Data Analysis Procedure

After the removal of duplicates, the citations were reviewed to identify the symptoms relevant to CR. Inclusion and exclusion criteria were applied to judge the eligibility of each citation in terms of its likelihood of describing CR. Citations mentioning the following terms, which refer to other diseases, were excluded: *Zhong feng*

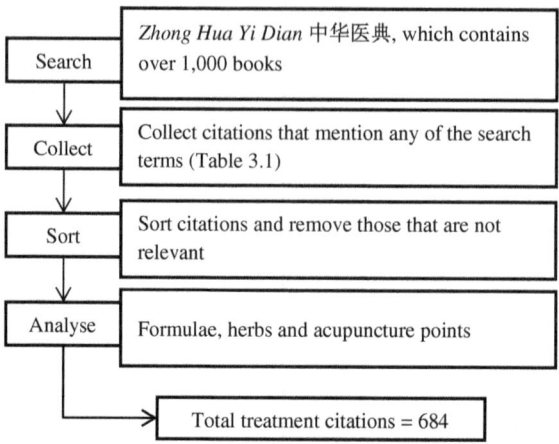

Fig. 3.1. Search process for classical literature citations.

中风 (stroke), *zhong* 肿 (swelling, possibly arthritis), *guan jie tong* 关节痛 (joint pain, possibly arthritis), *fa re* 发热 (fever, possibly arthritis), *shou chou chu* 手抽搐 (twitching, possibly Parkinson's disease), and *re* 热 (heat, possibly arthritis).

All relevant citations were further coded to find out whether they contained the following two groups of terms:

- Location terms: *Jian* 肩 (shoulder), *nao* 臑 (upper limb), *bo* 膊 (arm), *zhou* 肘 (elbow), *bi* (2) 臂 (arm), *wan* 腕 (wrist), *shou* 手 (hand), *zhang* 掌 (palm of hand), *zhi* 指 (finger), *jing* 颈 (neck) and *xiang* 项 (nape); and
- Representative symptom terms related to CR: *Teng* 疼 (pain), *tong* 痛 (pain), *ma* 麻 (numbness), *bu ren* 不仁 (numbness), *Bi* (1) 痹 (impediment disease or arthralgia) and *suan chu* 酸楚 (soreness).

Citations that described at least two location terms and any representative symptom terms were judged as "possible CR" citations. Citations that contained at least two location terms and pain symptoms (*teng* 疼 or *tong* 痛) were determined as "most likely CR" citations. All relevant citations were reviewed to identify the best descriptions of CR and its aetiology and pathogenesis.

Citations were separated for analysis if they contained multiple treatments. Where herbal ingredients for Chinese herbal medicine (CHM) formulae were not detailed in citations, the herbs were sought from other descriptions of the formula within the same book. If herb ingredients were not able to be identified from the same book, the ingredients were then cited from the *Zhong Yi Fang Ji Da Ci Dian* 中医方剂大辞典, which is one of the most comprehensive collections of CHM formulae. Descriptive statistical methods were applied to analyse the most frequently mentioned CHM formulae, herbal ingredients and acupuncture points in the classical literature.

Search Results

A total of 23,677 hits (instances) in the ZHYD were obtained by the 17 search terms and 8 combinations of terms (see Table 3.2). Not surprisingly, the term *bi* (2) 臂 produced the largest number of hits (9,996, 42.22%) because it is a general anatomy term meaning "arm" and is relevant to various conditions. The combination of *Bi* (1) 痹 and *xiang* 项, with the translated meaning of "impediment disease and nape", produced the second largest number of hits (2,582, 10.91%). Other combinations of terms that obtained more than 5% of the total instances include *tou tong* 头痛 and *bi* (2) 臂 (headache and arm, 2,107 hits, 8.90%), *Bi* (1) 痹 and *jian* 肩 (impediment disease and shoulder, 2,097, 8.86%) and *Bi* (1) 痹 and *bi* (2) 臂 (impediment disease and arm, 1,358, 5.74%). The search terms of *bo jing* 脖颈 and *jing jian tong* 颈肩痛 did not yield any results.

Citations Related to Cervical Radiculopathy

A total of 684 citations met the inclusion criteria and were considered "possible CR" citations. Sixty-nine citations that described relevant symptoms and aetiology/pathogenesis of this condition but without treatments were reviewed for summary.

Of the 684 Chinese medicine treatment citations, 627 were further judged as "most likely CR" citations because they described the most representative symptom "pain" in their texts. Among these 684

Table 3.2. Hit Frequency by Search Term and Combination

Pinyin	**Chinese Characters**	**Total Hit Frequency (*n*, %)**
Bi (2)	臂	9,996 (42.22)
Bi (1) and *xiang*	痹 and 项	2,582 (10.91)
Tou tong and *bi* (2)	头痛 and 臂	2,107 (8.90)
Bi (1) and *jian*	痹 and 肩	2,097 (8.86)
Bi (1) and *bi* (2)	痹 and 臂	1,358 (5.74)
Gu tong and *bi* (2)	骨痛 and 臂	923 (3.90)
Xiang tong	项痛	793 (3.35)
Bi (2) *tong*	臂痛	682 (2.88)
Xiang jiang	项强	675 (2.85)
Jing xiang	颈项	612 (2.58)
Jian bei tong	肩背痛	331 (1.40)
Gu bi (1) and *bi* (2)	骨痹 and 臂	302 (1.28)
Zhi jie tong	肢节痛	203 (0.86)
Xuan yun and *bi* (2) *tong*	眩晕 and 臂痛	162 (0.68)
Jian tong	肩痛	134 (0.57)
Shou ma	手麻	109 (0.46)
Bi (2) *jue*	臂厥	100 (0.42)
Shang zhi	上肢	72 (0.30)
Jing xiang tong	颈项痛	66 (0.28)
Tan zheng and *bi* (2)	痰症 and 臂	65 (0.46)
Shou tong	手痛	60 (0.25)
Xiang jin ji	项筋急	58 (0.24)
Bi (2) *teng*	臂疼	50 (0.21)
Xiang bei tong	项背痛	37 (0.16)
Jing jin ji	颈筋急	24 (0.10)
Ji bei tong	脊背痛	21 (0.09)
Jian bi (2) *tong*	肩臂痛	21 (0.09)
Shou teng tong	手疼痛	18 (0.08)
Bi (2) *bing*	臂病	8 (0.03)
Jing bi (1)	颈痹	4 (0.02)

Table 3.2. (*Continued*)

Pinyin	Chinese Characters	Total Hit Frequency (*n*, %)
Jian men	肩门	3 (0.01)
Xiang bi (2) tong	项臂痛	1 (<0.01)
Bi (2) zheng	臂症	1 (<0.01)
Jia ji tong	夹脊痛	1 (<0.01)
Xiang bi (1)	项痹	1 (<0.01)
Bo jing	脖颈	0
Jing jian tong	颈肩痛	0
Total		**23,677**

citations, 352 citations mentioned CHM as management for CR, 323 citations introduced acupuncture and related therapies, and 9 citations recommended other Chinese medicine therapies such as *daoyin* 导引 (a type of physical exercises involving *qigong* 气功) and massage.

Descriptions of Cervical Radiculopathy

In classical Chinese medicine literature, CR symptoms were commonly described under *Bi* (1) disease 痹证, which refers to a group of diseases manifesting local pain, soreness, heaviness, numbness or restricted mobility involving muscles, tendon, bones and joints.[17] In terms of typical symptoms, cervical spondylosis, rheumatic arthritis, rheumatoid arthritis, gout, spinal stenosis, etc., could possibly be included in *Bi* (1) disease 痹证. As a result, some descriptions of the aetiology and pathogenesis of *Bi* (1) disease 痹证 were likely referring to CR in past eras.

In history, the typical clinical manifestations of CR including shoulder and neck pain, arm pain and restricted upper limb mobility were mentioned in various classical literature. One of the earliest possible descriptions was obtained from the book *Huang Di Nei Jing* 黄帝内经 (474–221 BCE). In the *Ling Shu·Jing Mai Pian* 灵枢·经脉篇

section, the author described a series of symptoms of *jing bi* (1) 颈痹: "Inability to fully turn one's head, feeling stiffness and tension in one's shoulder as if being pulled by another person and suffering severe pain in the arm and shoulder 不可以顾, 肩似拔, 臑似折. The pain could occur in the chin, shoulder, arm (anterior and posterior), elbow or forearm 颔, 肩, 臑, 肘, 臂外后廉痛". Huang-Fu Mi 皇甫谧 in his book *Zhen Jiu Jia Yi Jing* 针灸甲乙经 (282 CE) stated that "the acupuncture point SI5 *Yanggu* 阳谷 could be used to manage patients' shoulder pain, inability to dress themselves, radial arm and wrist pain, and restricted mobility 肩痛, 不可自带衣, 臂腕外侧痛不举, 阳谷主之". These descriptions are consistent with the contemporary clinical understanding of CR.

Descriptions of the Aetiology of Cervical Radiculopathy

The earliest discussion of aetiology related to CR was from the *Huang Di Nei Jing* 黄帝内经. In the *Su Wen·Bi Lun* 素问·痹论 section, the authors wrote: "*Bi* (1) disease 痹证 (impediment disease or arthralgia) is generated by the combined invasion of wind, cold and dampness pathological factors. If the wind factor dominates, the pain migrates quickly. If the cold factor dominates, the pain tends to be severe. If the dampness factor dominates, the pain is often localised and does not migrate (风, 寒, 湿三气杂至, 合而为痹也. 其风气胜者为行痹, 其寒气胜者为痛痹, 湿气胜者为着痹也)". Gu Jing-Yuan 顾靖远 also described in his book *Gu Song Yuan Yi Jing* 顾松园医镜 (1718 CE) the pathogenesis of wind, cold and dampness that separately causes *Bi* (1) disease 痹证: "Pathogenic wind can attack the defence *qi* 卫气 of the human body, then induce *qi* stagnation to generate *Bi* (1) disease 痹证; pathogenic cold attacks the nutrients and Blood of the human body, then causes the skin to lose nutrient support and generates *Bi* (1) disease 痹证; pathogenic dampness invades the muscles and induces meridian blockages to cause *Bi* (1) disease 痹证 (有因风伤卫气, 气凝不行而致者, 有因寒伤荣血, 皮肤不荣而致者, 有因湿伤肌肉, 脉理不通而致者)". In general, the pathological factors of wind, cold and dampness were considered the main external causes that generate *Bi* (1) disease 痹证.

In classical Chinese medicine literature, internal causes were also considered pathological factors generating *Bi* (1) disease 痹证 and pain. Chen Wen-You 程文囿 in his book *Yi Shu* 医述 (1826 CE) noted that "the *yang ming* 阳明 meridians (the large intestine and stomach meridians) create the most *qi* among the 12 meridians in the human body, and that arm pain is mainly induced by diseases of the *yang ming* 阳明 meridians (阳明为十二经络之长, 臂痛赤当责之阳明)." and "when meridians lose sufficient nutritional support, internal wind occurs and causes stiffness of tendons, which can be treated by *Dong yuan shu jing tang* 东垣舒筋汤 and *Huo luo dan* 活络丹 (如营虚脉络失养, 风动筋急者… 当仿东垣舒筋汤之意, 佐以活络丹)". He also wrote that "*qi* deficiency in the *yang ming* 阳明 meridians could cause internal wind of the *jue yin* 厥阴 meridian to generate right shoulder pain and numbness. This *qi* 气 and nutrient deficiency syndrome of the *yang ming* 阳明 and *jue yin* 厥阴 meridians could be treated by CHM such as *gou qi* 枸杞, *dang gui shen* 当归身, *huang qi* 黄芪, *ling yang jiao* 羚羊角 and *sang zhi* 桑枝 (阳明气衰, 厥阴风动, 右肩痛麻者, 用枸杞, 归身, 黄芪, 羚角, 桑枝, 为阳明, 厥阴营气两虚主治)". In the *Zhang Shi Yi Tong* 张氏医通 (1695 CE), the author held a similar opinion on *Bi* (1) disease 痹证: "*Zhuo bi* (1) 着痹 manifests numbness as the main symptom and it does not migrate". As the *Huang Di Nei Jing* 黄帝内经 noted, "nutrient *qi* deficiency could cause (skin and muscle) numbness, while defensive *qi* deficiency could induce restricted mobility (of the body). When both nutrient *qi* and defensive *qi* are deficient, these symptoms could appear together (著痹者, 痹著不仁. 经曰, 营气虚则不仁, 卫气虚则不用, 营卫俱虚则, 不仁且不用)".

Phlegm was determined as another internal pathological factor likely related to CR. In the book *Wan Bing Hui Chun* 万病回春 (1587 CE), Gong Ting-Xian 龚廷贤 noted: "Phlegm could induce various symptoms including arm pain radiating to the shoulder and back, numbness of the hands and feet, and arthritis-like arm pain (或四肢筋骨疼痛, 或手足麻痹, 臂痛状若风湿, 皆痰所致)". The Japanese Chinese medicine practitioner Dan-bo-yuan-jian 丹波元坚 in his book *Za Bing Guang Yao* 杂病广要 (1853 CE) further suggested that "phlegm and retained fluid flowing into the limbs could generate a series of symptoms, including feeling pain and soreness in the arms, shoulder and back, lack of strength in the hand and numbness in the hands (臂连肩背酸痛, 两手软痹, 由痰饮流入四肢也)".

Traumatic injury was also mentioned to induce arm pain in classical literature. Chen Wen-You 程文囿 in the book *Yi Shu* 医述 (1826 CE) wrote that "arm pain could be induced by the invasion of wind, cold and dampness pathological factors, phlegm accumulation and *qi* stagnation or lifting heavy weights 臂为风寒湿所搏, 或痰流气滞, 或因提挈重物, 皆致臂痛". He also noted that "overexertion or a sedentary lifestyle of reading books or playing chess could generate spinal or back pain, which could be managed by *Bu zhong yi qi tang* 补中益气汤 or *Ba wei tang* 八味汤 plus *huang qi* 黄芪 (有因劳力或看书, 着棋久坐而致脊背痛者, 宜补中益气汤, 或八味汤加黄芪)". This is consistent with the current clinical understanding that inappropriate long-term overhead work and neck injuries are risk factors for CR.

Chinese Herbal Medicine

There were 352 CHM treatment citations obtained from 111 books. The book that produced the largest number of citations was the *Za Bing Guang Yao* 杂病广要 (1853 CE, *n* = 35). Other books that yielded more than 15 citations included the *Pu Ji Fang* 普济方 (1406 CE, *n* = 27), *Feng Shi Zhi Yao* 奉时旨要 (1830 CE, *n* = 15) and *Zheng Zhi Zhun Sheng·Za Bing* 证治准绳·杂病 (1602 CE, *n* = 15). Oral CHM treatments were mentioned in most of the included citations (350 citations), while topical formulae were only introduced in two citations: One introduced a method of treating CR with a CHM topical warming application, and the other applied a hot medicinal compress therapy.

Frequency of Treatment Citations by Dynasty

The included CHM treatment citations were obtained from the books published from the Tang and Five dynasties (618–960 CE) to the Minguo 民国/Republic of China (1912–1949 CE) (Table 3.3). The vast majority of citations were published in the Ming dynasty (1369–1644

Table 3.3. Dynastic Distribution of Treatment Citations

Dynasty	No. of Citations
Tang and 5 Dynasties (618–960 CE)	1
Song and Jin Dynasties (961–1271 CE)	20
Yuan Dynasty (1272–1368 CE)	4
Ming Dynasty (1369–1644 CE)	123
Qing Dynasty (1645–1911 CE)	198
Min Guo/Republic of China (1912–1949 CE)	6
Total	**352**

CE) and Qing dynasty (1645–1911 CE) (321 citations, 91.2%), possibly due to the advancing printing techniques during these eras. The earliest citation describing CHM treatment was from the *Xian Shou Li Shang Xu Duan Mi Fang* 仙授理伤续断秘方 (846 CE). It mentioned that "*Da huo xue dan* 大活血丹 can be used to manage various health conditions including injuries of tendons, diseases generated by wind pathogen, paralysis, numbness of limbs and feeling of pain, which were likely related to CR (大活血丹, 治扑损伤折, 骨碎筋伤, 疼痛浮肿, 腹有瘀血, 灌注四肢, 烦满不安; 痈疽发背, 筋肉坏烂; 诸般风疾, 左瘫右痪, 手足顽麻; 妇人血风诸疾, 产后败血不行, 流入四肢, 头面浮肿, 血气疼痛; 浑身疼痹; 经脉湛浊, 风痨发动, 百节酸疼, 并宜服之)". The most recent citation was a case report from the *Wang Zhong Qi Yi An* 王仲奇医案 (1945 CE). The author described a patient complaining of right shoulder pain and stiffness and tension in the limbs, restricted joint mobility and difficulties in raising arms (右肩髃疼痛, 筋骨拘急, 机关不利, 臂难上举). He quoted Zhang Zhong-Jing's 张仲景 discussion that "restricted arm mobility was a sort of *Bi* (1) disease 痹证" and prescribed a formula for this patient under the principle of activating the Blood and soothing the tendons.

Treatment with Oral Chinese Herbal Medicine

In total, 350 possible CR citations introduced oral CHM treatments. A subset of 321 citations described the most typical pain (*teng/tong* 疼/痛)

symptom and was considered most likely related to CR. The oral formulae and herbs mentioned in these citations were analysed for the total number possible, and for the subset most likely to be CR pools.

Most Frequent Oral Formulae in Citations Possibly Related to Cervical Radiculopathy

A total of 162 oral formulae were identified from the 350 citations. More than half of the included formulae were unnamed (*n* = 84, 51.9%). Most formulae contained multiple herbal ingredients, while only seven were identified as single-herb formulae. Twelve formulae were mentioned in more than five citations and are presented in Table 3.4. Formulae with different names were pooled together for

Table 3.4. Most Frequent Formulae for Oral Use in Citations Possibly Related to Cervical Radiculopathy

Formula Name	Herb Ingredients	No. of Citations (*n*)
Fu ling wan/Zhi mi fu ling wan/Zhi mi wan 茯苓丸/指迷茯苓丸/指迷丸	*Fu ling* 茯苓, *zhi ke* 枳壳, *ban xia* 半夏, *mang xiao* 芒硝, and *sheng jiang* 生姜 (*Huo Ren Shi Zheng Fang Hou Ji* 活人事证方后集, 1216 CE)	47
Juan bi tang/Juan bi tang jia jian 蠲痹汤/蠲痹汤加减	*Dang gui* 当归, *chi shao* 赤芍, *huang qi* 黄芪, *fang feng* 防风, *pian jiang huang* 片姜黄, *qiang huo* 羌活, *zhi gan cao* 炙甘草, *sheng jiang* 生姜, and *da zhao* 大枣 (*Ren Zhai Zhi Zhi Fang Lun* 仁斋直指方论, 1264 CE)	26
Er chen tang/Er chen tang jia jian 二陈汤/二陈汤加减	*Ban xia* 半夏, *chen pi* 陈皮, *gan cao* 甘草, *fu ling* 茯苓, and *pian jiang huang* 片姜黄 (*Ren Zhai Zhi Zhi Fang Lun* 仁斋直指方论, 1264 CE)	15
Dao tan tang/Dao tan tang jia jian 导痰汤/导痰汤加减	*Ban xia* 半夏, *chen pi* 陈皮, *fu ling* 茯苓, *gan cao* 甘草, *tian nan xing* 天南星, *zhi shi* 枳实, *mu xiang* 木香, and *jiang huang* 姜黄 (*Zheng Zhi Zhun Sheng* 证治准绳, 1604 CE)	15

Table 3.4. (*Continued*)

Formula Name	Herb Ingredients	No. of Citations (*n*)
Kong xian dan/Kong xian dan jia jian 控涎丹/控涎丹加减	*Gan sui* 甘遂, *jing da ji* 京大戟, *jie zi* 芥子, *mu bie zi* 木鳖子, and *rou gui* 肉桂 (*Yi Xue Zheng Zhuan* 医学正传, 1515 CE)	13
Wu ji san/Wu ji san jia jian 五积散/五积散加减	*Bai zhi* 白芷, *zhi ke* 枳壳, *ma huang* 麻黄, *cang zhu* 苍术, *gan jiang* 干姜, *jie geng* 桔梗, *hou po* 厚朴, *gan cao* 甘草, *fu ling* 茯苓, *dang gui* 当归, *rou gui* 肉桂, *chuan xiong* 川芎, *shao yao* 芍药, *ban xia* 半夏, *chen pi* 陈皮, *chai hu* 柴胡, *jie geng* 桔梗, *ren shen* 人参, *qian hu* 前胡, *qiang huo* 羌活, *du huo* 独活, *mu gua* 木瓜, and *niu xi* 牛膝 (*Xiao Zhu Fu Ren Liang Fang* 校注妇人良方, 1558 CE)	12
Wu yao shun qi san/ Wu yao shun qi san jia jian 乌药顺气散/ 乌药顺气散加减	*Wu yao* 乌药, *chen pi* 陈皮, *ma huang* 麻黄, *zhi ke* 枳壳, *jie geng* 桔梗, *bai zhi* 白芷, *chuan xiong* 川芎, *jiang chan* 僵蚕, *gan jiang* 干姜, *gan cao* 甘草, *gui zhi* 桂枝, *cang zhu* 苍术, *qiang huo* 羌活, *fang feng* 防风, and *gan jiang* 干姜 (*Za Bing Zhi Li* 杂病治例, 1479 CE)	8
San bi tang 三痹汤	*Xu duan* 续断, *du zhong* 杜仲, *fang feng* 防风, *rou gui* 肉桂, *xi xin* 细辛, *ren shen* 人参, *fu ling* 茯苓, *dang gui* 当归, *bai shao* 白芍, *gan cao* 甘草, *qin jiao* 秦艽, *sheng di* 生地, *chuan xiong* 川芎, *du huo* 独活, *huang qi* 黄芪, *chuan niu xi* 川牛膝, and *sheng jiang* 生姜, *da zhao* 大枣 (*Fu Ren Da Quan Liang Fang* 妇人大全良方, 1237 CE)	6
Shu jing tang 舒筋汤	*Qiang huo* 羌活, *gan cao* 甘草, *dang gui* 当归, *jiang huang* 姜黄, *bai zhu* 白术, *chi shao* 赤芍, *hai tong pi* 海桐皮, and *sheng jiang* 生姜 (*Pu Ji Fang* 普济方, 1406 CE)	6
Gun tan wan 滚痰丸	*Da huang* 大黄, *huang qin* 黄芩, *chen xiang* 沉香, *qing meng shi* 青礞石, and *zhu sha* 朱砂 (*Gu Jin Yi Tong Da Quan* 古今医统大全, 1556 CE)	5

(*Continued*)

Table 3.4. (*Continued*)

Formula Name	Herb Ingredients	No. of Citations (*n*)
Shen xiao huang qi tang 神效黄芪汤	*Huang qi* 黄芪, *ren shen* 人参, *zhi gan cao* 炙甘草, *man jing zi* 蔓荆子, *bai shao* 白芍, and *ju pi* 菊皮 (*Pu Ji Fang* 普济方, 1406 CE)	5
Qiang huo sheng shi tang 羌活胜湿汤	*Qiang huo* 羌活, *du huo* 独活, *zhi gan cao* 炙甘草, *gao ben* 藁本, *fang feng* 防风, *chuan xiong* 川芎, and *man jing zi* 蔓荆子 (*Bao Ming Ge Kuo* 保命歌括, 1567 CE)	5

Note: The use of some herbs/ingredients may be restricted in some countries. For example, the herbs *ma huang* 麻黄 and *zhu sha* 朱砂 can be toxic. Readers are advised to comply with relevant regulations.

frequency analysis if they originated from the same basic formula and shared similar ingredients. Herbal ingredients were obtained from the earliest citation if variants were seen under the same formula name.

The most frequently cited formula was *Fu ling wan/Zhi mi fu ling wan/Zhi mi wan* 茯苓丸/指迷茯苓丸/指迷丸, which was obtained from 47 citations. The earliest citation mentioning this formula was from the *Huo Ren Shi Zheng Fang Hou Ji* 活人事证方后集 (1216 CE). The author, Liu Xin-Fu 刘信甫, wrote that "*Fu ling wan* 茯苓丸 can be used to dispel phlegm and was originally for managing arm pain (治痰茯苓丸, 本治臂痛)". Herbal ingredients in this formula have the function of clearing dampness, regulating *qi* 气 to resolve phlegm. In this book the author also referenced the aetiology discussion of arm pain from *Zhi mi fang* 指迷方: "Phlegm retention (*fu tan* 伏痰) in the abdomen could generate arm pain by restraining Spleen *qi* 气. When *qi* stagnation happens, *qi* cannot flow downwards normally and refluxes upwards, then attacks the arms, which are dominated by the Spleen. This type of arm pain is related to the syndrome of phlegm and could be effectively managed by phlegm-dispelling treatments (由伏痰在内, 中脘停滞, 脾气不流行, 上与气搏, 四肢属脾, 滞而气不下, 故上行攻臂, 其脉沉细者是也, 后人谓此臂痛乃痰证也, 用以治痰无不效者)". Many commonly cited formulae such as *Er chen tang/Er chen tang jia jian* 二陈汤/二陈汤加减, *Dao tan tang/Dao tan tang jia jian*

导痰汤/导痰汤加减, *Kong xian dan/Kong xian dan jia jian* 控涎丹/控涎丹加减, *Wu ji san/Wu ji san jia jian* 五积散/五积散加减 and *Gun tan wan* 滚痰丸 carried similar functions of draining dampness and resolving phlegm. This is consistent with contemporary understanding from Chinese medicine textbooks and guidelines that dampness and phlegm are the two main pathogens of CR (see Chap. 2).

Other frequently mentioned formulae have different functions. *Juan bi tang/Juan bi tang jia jian* 蠲痹汤/蠲痹汤加减, *Qiang huo sheng shi tang* 羌活胜湿汤 and *Shu jing tang* 舒筋汤 have the functions of dispelling wind and dampness, resolving impediment and alleviating pain. *Juan bi tang/Juan bi tang jia jian* 蠲痹汤/蠲痹汤加减 and *Qiang huo sheng shi tang* 羌活胜湿汤 are both recommended by contemporary guidelines and textbooks for treating the syndrome of wind and cold blocking meridians. *San bi tang* 三痹汤 has the functions of nourishing *qi* 气 and Blood, expelling cold and wind, and draining dampness; *Wu yao shun qi san/Wu yao shun qi san jia jian* 乌药顺气散/乌药顺气散加减 carries the function of dispelling wind to resolve impediment; *Shen xiao huang qi tang* 神效黄芪汤 tonifies *qi*, soothes the Liver and expels wind. In summary, expelling wind is the key function of these formulae, which is also consistent with current knowledge that wind is one of the pathological factors generating CR.

Most Frequent Herbs for Oral Use in Citations Possibly Related to Cervical Radiculopathy

A total of 246 oral herbal ingredients were obtained from the included formulae. The most commonly reported herbs (being used in more than 20 formulae) are presented in Table 3.5. The key clinical function of these herbs is to resolve impediment and they can be sorted into seven categories:

- Drain dampness and expel phlegm to resolve impediment: *Fu ling* 茯苓, *ban xia* 半夏, *bai zhu* 白术 and *cang zhu* 苍术;
- Expel wind and cold to resolve impediment and alleviate pain: *Qiang huo* 羌活, *fang feng* 防风, *chuan xiong* 川芎, *sheng jiang* 生姜, *bai zhi* 白芷 and *ma huang* 麻黄;

Table 3.5. Most Frequent Oral Herbs in Citations Possibly Related to Cervical Radiculopathy

Herb Name	Scientific Name	No. of Citations (*n*)
Gan cao 甘草	1. *Glycyrrhiza uralensis* Fish. 2. *Glycyrrhiza inflata* Bat. 3. *Glycyrrhiza glabra* L.	195
Fu ling 茯苓	*Poria cocos* (Schw.) Wolf.	166
Ban xia 半夏	*Pinellia ternata* (Thunb.) Breit.	147
Dang gui 当归	*Angelica sinensis* (Oliv.) Diels	126
Sheng jiang/Gan jiang 生姜/干姜	*Zingiber officinale* Rosc.	124 (84/40)
Shao yao/Chi shao/Bai shao 芍药/赤芍/白芍	1. *Paeonia lactiflora* Pall. 2. *Paeonia veitchii* Lynch.	111 (42/27/40)
Qiang huo 羌活	1. *Notopterygium incisum* Ting ex H.T. Chang 2. *Notopterygium franchetii* H. de Boiss.	104
Zhi ke 枳壳	*Citrus aurantium* L.	100
Chen pi 陈皮	*Citrus reticulata* Blanco.	96
Fang feng 防风	*Saposhnikovia divaricata* (Turcz.) Schischk.	87
Chuan xiong 川芎	*Ligusticum chuanxiong* Hort.	74
Huang qi 黄芪	1. *Astragalus membranaceus* (Fisch.) Bge. var. mongholicus (Bge.) Hsiao 2. *Astragalus membranaceus* (Fisch.) Bge.	64
Rou gui 肉桂	*Cinnamomum cassia* Presl	60
Mang xiao 芒硝	Hydrated sodium sulfate	57
Bai zhu 白术	*Atractylodes macrocephala* Koidz.	54
Cang zhu 苍术	1. *Atractylodes lancea* (Thunb.) DC. 2. *Atractylodes chinensis* (DC.) Koidz.	52
Jiang huang 姜黄	*Curcuma longa* L.	52
Ren shen 人参	*Panax ginseng* C.A. Mey.	49

Table 3.5. (*Continued*)

Herb Name	Scientific Name	No. of Citations (*n*)
Bai zhi 白芷	1. *Angelica dahurica* (Fisch. ex Hoffm.) Benth. et Hook. f. 2. *Angelica dahurica* (Fisch. ex Hoffm.) Benth. et Hook. f. var. formosana (Boiss.) Shan et Yuan	46
Ma huang 麻黄	1. *Ephedra sinica* Stapf 2. *Ephedra equisetina* Bge. 3. *Ephedra intermedia* Schrenk et C.A. Mey.	42

- Regulate *qi* to resolve impediment and alleviate pain: *Zhi ke* 枳壳, *chen pi* 陈皮 and *jiang huang* 姜黄;
- Tonify *qi* and warm meridians to resolve impediment: *Gan cao* 甘草, *huang qi* 黄芪 and *ren shen* 人参;
- Tonify Blood and *yin* to resolve impediment: *Dang gui* 当归 and *shao yao* 芍药;
- Warm meridians and expel cold to resolve impediment and alleviate pain: *Rou gui* 肉桂; and
- Clear damp-heat and reduce swelling and pain: *Mang xiao* 芒硝.

Not surprisingly, the most frequent herb for oral use was found to be *gan cao* 甘草. In Chinese medicine practice, *gan cao* 甘草 is widely used for harmonising other herbs in formulations, which is likely to contribute to its high frequency in classical books. *Gan cao* 甘草 also has the function to tonify *qi* and nourish the Spleen, relieve the tension of tendons and alleviate pain. It is beneficial for treating CR generated by Spleen and *qi* deficiency.

Fu ling 茯苓 and *ban xia* 半夏, both carrying the clinical functions of draining dampness and expelling phlegm, were found to be the second and third most commonly cited herbs among the included formulae. These two herbs are also the key ingredients in several of the most frequently reported formulae including *Fu ling wan/Zhi mi fu ling wan/Zhi mi wan* 茯苓丸/指迷茯苓丸/指迷丸, *Er chen tang/Er chen tang jia jian* 二陈汤/二陈汤加减 and *Dao tan tang/Dao tan tang jia jian* 导痰汤/导痰汤加减. In contemporary Chinese medicine guidelines,[18] *Ban xia bai zhu tian ma tang* 半夏白术天麻汤 with *fu ling* 茯苓 and *ban xia* 半夏 as main ingredients are recommended for managing CR in relation to phlegm and dampness blocking the meridian syndrome. This suggests their importance in managing CR.

Most Frequent Oral Formulae in Most Likely Cervical Radiculopathy Citations

Among the 350 citations describing oral CHM treatments, the majority (321 citations, 91.7%) were further judged "most likely" to be CR citations because they mentioned pain as a symptom. This may contribute to similar lists of the most frequent oral formulae and herbs summarised from both the "most likely" and "possible" CR citation pools.

A total of 150 formulae were obtained from the included citations and half of these were unnamed formulae (*n* = 75, 50.0%). Twelve formulae were mentioned in more than four citations (Table 3.6). Ten of the most frequently reported oral formulae were

Table 3.6. Most Frequent Oral Formulae in Most Likely Cervical Radiculopathy Citations

Formula Name	Herb Ingredients	No. of Citations (*n*)
Fu ling wan/Zhi mi fu ling wan/Zhi mi wan 茯苓丸/指迷茯苓丸/指迷丸	*Fu ling* 茯苓, *zhi ke* 枳壳, *ban xia* 半夏, mang xiao 芒硝, and sheng jiang 生姜 (*Huo Ren Shi Zheng Fang Hou Ji* 活人事证方后集, 1216 CE)	45
Juan bi tang/Juan bi tang jia jian 蠲痹汤/蠲痹汤加减	Dang gui 当归, *chi shao* 赤芍, *huang qi* 黄芪, *fang feng* 防风, *pian jiang huang* 片姜黄, *qiang huo* 羌活, *zhi gan cao* 炙甘草, *sheng jiang* 生姜, and *da zhao* 大枣 (*Ren Zhai Zhi Zhi Fang Lun* 仁斋直指方论, 1264 CE)	26

Table 3.6. (*Continued*)

Formula Name	Herb Ingredients	No. of Citations (*n*)
Er chen tang/Er chen tang jia jian 二陈汤/二陈汤加减	*Ban xia* 半夏, *chen pi* 陈皮, *gan cao* 甘草, *fu ling* 茯苓, and *pian jiang huang* 片姜黄 (*Ren Zhai Zhi Zhi Fang Lun* 仁斋直指方论, 1264 CE)	14
Dao tan tang/ Dao tan tang jia jian 导痰汤/导痰汤加减	*Ban xia* 半夏, *chen pi* 陈皮, *fu ling* 茯苓, *gan cao* 甘草, *tian nan xing* 天南星, *zhi shi* 枳实, *mu xiang* 木香, and *jiang huang* 姜黄 (*Zheng Zhi Zhun Sheng* 证治准绳, 1604 CE)	14
Kong xian dan/ Kong xian dan jia jian 控涎丹/控涎丹加减	*Gan sui* 甘遂, *jing da ji* 京大戟, *jie zi* 芥子, *mu bie zi* 木鳖子, and *rou gui* 肉桂 (*Yi Xue Zheng Zhuan* 医学正传, 1515 CE)	13
Wu ji san/Wu ji san jia jian 五积散/五积散加减	*Bai zhi* 白芷, *zhi ke* 枳壳, *ma huang* 麻黄, *cang zhu* 苍术, *gan jiang* 干姜, *jie geng* 桔梗, *hou po* 厚朴, *gan cao* 甘草, *fu ling* 茯苓, *dang gui* 当归, *rou gui* 肉桂, *chuan xiong* 川芎, *shao yao* 芍药, *ban xia* 半夏, *chen pi* 陈皮, *chai hu* 柴胡, *jie geng* 桔梗, *ren shen* 人参, *qian hu* 前胡, *qiang huo* 羌活, *du huo* 独活, *mu gua* 木瓜, and *niu xi* 牛膝 (*Xiao Zhu Fu Ren Liang Fang* 校注妇人良方, 1558 CE)	11
Wu yao shun qi san/Wu yao shun qi san jia jian 乌药顺气散/乌药顺气散加减	*Wu yao* 乌药, *chen pi* 陈皮, *ma huang* 麻黄, *zhi ke* 枳壳, *jie geng* 桔梗, *bai zhi* 白芷, *chuan xiong* 川芎, *jiang chan* 僵蚕, *gan jiang* 干姜, *gan cao* 甘草, *gui zhi* 桂枝, *cang zhu* 苍术, *qiang huo* 羌活, *fang feng* 防风, and *gan jiang* 干姜 (*Za Bing Zhi Li* 杂病治例, 1479 CE)	8
Shu jing tang 舒筋汤	*Qiang huo* 羌活, *gan cao* 甘草, *dang gui* 当归, *jiang huang* 姜黄, *bai zhu* 白术, *chi shao* 赤芍, *hai tong pi* 海桐皮, and *sheng jiang* 生姜 (*Pu Ji Fang* 普济方, 1406 CE)	6
Gun tan wan 滚痰丸	*Da huang* 大黄, *huang qin* 黄芩, *chen xiang* 沉香, *qing meng shi* 青礞石, and *zhu sha* 朱砂 (*Gu Jin Yi Tong Da Quan* 古今医统大全, 1556 CE)	5

(*Continued*)

Table 3.6. (*Continued*)

Formula Name	Herb Ingredients	No. of Citations (*n*)
Qiang huo sheng shi tang 羌活胜湿汤	*Qiang huo* 羌活, *du huo* 独活, *zhi gan cao* 炙甘草, *gao ben* 藁本, *fang feng* 防风, *chuan xiong* 川芎, and *man jing zi* 蔓荆子 (*Bao Ming Ge Kuo* 保命歌括, 1567 CE)	5
Ren shen san 人参散	*Ren shen* 人参, *bie jia* 鳖甲, *ling yang jiao* 羚羊角, *chi fu ling* 赤茯苓, *zhi mu* 知母, *chai hu* 柴胡, *di gu pi* 地骨皮, *zhi ke* 枳壳, *niu xi* 牛膝, *chi shao* 赤芍, *sheng di* 生地, *mu dan pi* 牡丹皮, *da huang* 大黄, *bai bu* 百部, *bei mu* 贝母, *huang qin* 黄芩, *gua lou gen* 栝蒌根, *dang gui* 当归, *tao ren* 桃仁, *cao dou kou* 草豆蔻, *an xi xiang* 安息香, *mang xiao* 芒硝, *zhi gan cao* 炙甘草, *zi wan* 紫菀, *mai dong* 麦冬, *tian men dong* 天门冬, and *tian ling gai* 天灵盖 (*Tai Ping Sheng Hui Fang* 太平圣惠方, 992 CE)	4
Tong qi fang feng tang 通气防风汤	*Qiang huo* 羌活, *du huo* 独活, *gao ben* 藁本, *fang feng* 防风, *gan cao* 甘草, *chuan xiong* 川芎, and *jing jie* 荆芥 (*Bao Ming Ge Kuo* 保命歌括, 1567 CE)	4

Note: The use of some herbs/ingredients may be restricted in some countries. For example, the herbs *ma huang* 麻黄 and *zhu sha* 朱砂 can be toxic. Readers are advised to comply with the relevant regulations.

also listed with high frequency in the total "possible CR" pool: *Fu ling wan/Zhi mi fu ling wan/Zhi mi wan* 茯苓丸/指迷茯苓丸/指迷丸, *Juan bi tang/Juan bi tang jia jian* 蠲痹汤/蠲痹汤加减, *Er chen tang/Er chen tang jia jian* 二陈汤/二陈汤加减, *Dao tan tang/Dao tan tang jia jian* 导痰汤/导痰汤加减, *Kong xian dan/Kong xian dan jia jian* 控涎丹/控涎丹加减, *Wu ji san/Wu ji san jia jian* 五积散/五积散加减, *Wu yao shun qi san/Wu yao shun qi san jia jian* 乌药顺气散/乌药顺气散加减, *Shu jing tang* 舒筋汤, *Gun tan wan* 滚痰丸 and *Qiang huo sheng shi tang* 羌活胜湿汤.

Ren shen san 人参散 and *Tong qi fang feng tang* 通气防风汤, the remaining two formulae, were found exclusively in the "most likely

CR" citations pool. Similar to the other most cited formulae, the key function of these two formulae is to resolve impediment. *Ren shen san* 人参散, first cited in the *Tai Ping Sheng Hui Fang* 太平圣惠方 (992 CE), has the function of tonifying *qi* and nourishing *yin* to resolve impediment. It can be used for managing various conditions including arm pain. *Tong qi fang feng tang* 通气防风汤 has the function of dispelling wind to resolve impediment and was historically widely used for managing shoulder and back pain possibly related to CR. In the book *Bao Ming Ge Kuo* 保命歌括 (1567 CE), the author stated that "*qi* stagnation and blocking of the Hand-*Taiyang* meridian could generate shoulder and back pain with restricted neck mobility, and could be managed by *Tong qi fang feng tang* 通气防风汤 (通气 防风汤 治肩背痛不可回顾者，此手太阳气郁而不行也)".

Most Frequent Herbs for Oral Use in Most Likely Cervical Radiculopathy Citations

A total of 238 herbal ingredients were identified from the "most likely CR" citations. The most frequently mentioned oral herbs are listed in Table 3.7. These most frequent herbs from the "most likely CR" citations were identical to those listed in the "possible CR" pool.

Table 3.7. Most Frequent Oral Herbs in Most Likely Cervical Radiculopathy Citations

Herb Name	Scientific Name	No. of Citations (*n*)
Gan cao 甘草	1. *Glycyrrhiza uralensis* Fish. 2. *Glycyrrhiza inflata* Bat. 3. *Glycyrrhiza glabra* L.	169
Fu ling 茯苓	*Poria cocos* (Schw.) Wolf.	153
Ban xia 半夏	*Pinellia ternata* (Thunb.) Breit.	137
Sheng jiang/Gan jiang 生姜/干姜	*Zingiber officinale* Rosc.	117
Dang gui 当归	*Angelica sinensis* (Oliv.) Diels	114

(Continued)

Table 3.7. (*Continued*)

Herb Name	Scientific Name	No. of Citations (*n*)
Qiang huo 羌活	1. *Notopterygium incisum* Ting ex H.T. Chang 2. *Notopterygium franchetii* H. de Boiss.	101
Shao yao/Chi shao/ Bai shao 芍药/赤芍/白芍	*Paeonia lactiflora* Pall.	96
Zhi ke 枳壳	*Citrus aurantium* L.	95
Chen pi 陈皮	*Citrus reticulata* Blanco	84
Fang feng 防风	*Saposhnikovia divaricata* (Turcz.) Schischk.	79
Chuan xiong 川芎	*Ligusticum chuanxiong* Hort.	69
Mang xiao 芒硝	Hydrated sodium sulfate	53
Rou gui 肉桂	*Cinnamomum cassia* Presl	53
Huang qi 黄芪	1. *Astragalus membranaceus* (Fisch.) Bge. var. mongholicus (Bge.) Hsiao 2. *Astragalus membranaceus* (Fisch.) Bge.	50
Bai zhu 白术	*Atractylodes macrocephala* Koidz.	50
Jiang huang 姜黄	*Curcuma longa* L.	50
Cang zhu 苍术	1. *Atractylodes lancea* (Thunb.) DC. 2. *Atractylodes chinensis* (DC.) Koidz.	47
Bai zhi 白芷	1. *Angelica dahurica* (Fisch. ex Hoffm.) Benth. et Hook. f. 2. *Angelica dahurica* (Fisch. ex Hoffm.) Benth. et Hook. f. var. formosana (Boiss.) Shan et Yuan	43
Ma huang 麻黄	1. *Ephedra sinica* Stapf 2. *Ephedra equisetina* Bge. 3. *Ephedra intermedia* Schrenk et C.A. Mey.	38
Ren shen 人参	1. *Panax ginseng* C.A. Mey.	37

Note: The use of some herbs/ingredients may be restricted in some countries. For example, the herbs *ma huang* 麻黄 can be toxic. Readers are advised to comply with the relevant regulations.

Treatment with Topical Chinese Herbal Medicine

Topical CHM treatments were described in two "most likely CR" citations. Unlike oral CHM management, the limited number suggests that topical CHM application might not have been historically popular for CR.

In the book *Bian Que Xin Shu* 扁鹊心书 (1146 CE), the author introduced a topical warming application mixture of *cao wu* 草乌, flour and vinegar to painful points for mild *Bi* (1) disease 痹证 including arm pain and stiffness and tension of the elbow (痹病, 风寒湿三气合而为痹, 走注疼痛, 或臂腰足膝拘挛, 两肘牵急, 乃寒邪凑于分肉之间也, 方书谓之白虎历节风 ... 若轻者不必灸, 用草乌末二两、白面二钱, 醋调熬成稀糊, 摊白布上, 乘热贴患处, 一宿而愈). In *Pu Ji Fang* 普济方 (1406 CE), while a hot medicinal compress therapy was recommended for arm and lower back pain, a powdered mixture of *dang gui* 当归, *fang feng* 防风, *gou ji* 狗脊, *gu bu sui* 骨碎补, *gao ben* 藁本, *xi xin* 细辛, *chi shao* 赤芍, *zi ran tong* 自然铜, *rou gui* 肉桂, *bi xie* 萆薢, and hot salt was prepared in a cloth bag, which was then used to press and rub the diseased area.

Discussion of Chinese Herbal Medicine for Cervical Radiculopathy

In our systematic review of the classical Chinese medicine literature evidence obtained from the ZHYD, oral CHM appeared to be a common therapy for symptoms related to CR. *Fu ling wan/Zhi mi fu ling wan/Zhi mi wan* 茯苓丸/指迷茯苓丸/指迷丸 was found to be the most frequently mentioned formula. Its herbal ingredients are formulated to drain dampness and resolve retention of the pathological factor phlegm to alleviate arm pain. The clinical function of this formula is consistent with the contemporary guideline recommending Modified *Ban xia bai zhu tian ma tang* 半夏白术天麻汤加减 for managing the syndrome of phlegm and dampness blocking meridians.

The two most frequently cited formulae — *Juan bi tang/Juan bi tang jia jian* 蠲痹汤/蠲痹汤加减 and *Qiang huo sheng shi tang* 羌活

胜湿汤 — in the citations judged most likely to be CR continue to be used in contemporary clinical Chinese medicine practice with guideline recommendations.[18] Both these formulae can be selected for treating the syndrome of wind and cold blocking meridians, as they have the function of dispelling the pathogens, resolving impediment and alleviating pain.

It should be noted that *ma huang* 麻黄, which was found to be one of the most commonly cited herbs in the classical literature most likely related to CR, might be restricted in some countries. In Australia, *ma huang* (ephedra spp.) has been listed as a prescription-only medicine and must be used under state and territory legislation.[19] Traditionally, *ma huang* has been categorised as an exterior-releasing medicinal that carries the functions of expelling wind and cold pathogens, and releasing the exterior. It could be used for managing CR identified as the "wind and cold blocking meridian syndrome". Contemporary guidelines recommend other herbs as replacements, such as *qiang huo* 羌活, *fang feng* 防风 and *chuang xiong* 川芎, which have similar expelling wind and cold functions to *ma huang* for CR.

Zhu sha 朱砂, an ingredient found in the most frequently mentioned formula *Gun tan wan* 滚痰丸 from the total pool, is also restricted by many countries due to its toxic active chemical compound, mercuric sulphide. In Australia, this has been listed as a Schedule 7 medicinal (dangerous poison).[19] *Zhu sha* is categorised as a settling tranquillising medicinal ingredient in CHM. It might be useful for treating phlegm-fire harassing the Heart spirit when formulated with other phlegm-expelling herbs in *Gun tan wan* 滚痰丸. In managing CR, *zhu sha* could be replaced by other non-toxic tranquillising ingredients such as *long gu* 龙骨 and *mu li* 牡蛎 in clinical practice.

Topical CHM therapies were found to be infrequently mentioned in classical Chinese medicine literature. Management, including topical herbal application and hot medicinal compress therapy, was introduced. This may suggest that oral Chinese medicine therapies were predominant management for CR in past eras.

Acupuncture and Related Therapies

A total of 323 citations describing acupuncture and related therapies were obtained from 42 books. The *Zhen Jiu Zi Sheng Jing* 针灸资生经 (1220 CE) was found to produce the largest number of citations (*n* = 67). Other books that yielded more than 20 citations included: *Pu Ji Fang·Zhen Jiu* 普济方·针灸 (1406 CE, 58 citations), *Zhen Jiu Jia Yi Jing* 针灸甲乙经 (282 CE, 36 citations) and *Zhen Jiu Da Cheng* 针灸大成 (1601 CE, 21 citations).

Frequency of Treatment Citations by Dynasty

The included citations were found in books published from the Jin 晋 dynasty (266–420 CE) to the Min Guo 民国/Republic of China period (1912–1949 CE) (Table 3.8). Books published during the Ming dynasty (1369–1644 CE) contributed the largest number of citations (*n* = 151, 46.7%). One possible reason was that two books, the *Pu Ji Fang·Zhen Jiu* 普济方·针灸 and *Zhen Jiu Da Cheng* 针灸大成 (1601 CE), producing the largest numbers of citations, were published during this period. The earliest citations were obtained from the *Zhen Jiu Jia Yi Jing* 针灸甲乙经. In this book, the author, Huangfu Mi 皇甫谧, listed a variety of acupuncture points for treating different clinical manifestations that related to CR. For example, "SI11 *Tianzong* 天宗

Table 3.8. Dynastic Distribution of Treatment Citations

Dynasty	No. of Citations
Before Tang Dynasty (before 618 CE)	37
Tang and 5 Dynasties (618–960 CE)	10
Song and Jin Dynasties (961–1271 CE)	68
Ming Dynasty (1369–1644 CE)	151
Qing Dynasty (1645–1911 CE)	45
Minguo/Republic of China (1912–1949 CE)	7
Total	**323**

can be used to treat those feeling a heavy weight on their shoulders and pain in their arms and elbows with restricted mobility (肩重肘臂痛, 不可举, 天宗主之)", while "LI12 *Zhouliao* 肘髎 can be selected for managing the feeling of soreness and a heavy weight on one's shoulder and elbow, arm pain and difficulty in flexion and extension (肩肘节酸重, 臂痛, 不可屈伸, 肘窌主之)". The latest citation was found in the book *Jin Zhen Mi Chuan* 金针秘传 (1937 CE). The author detailed a case report of left arm pain radiating to the hand. After three days of acupuncture treatment on the point LI11 *Quchi* 曲池, the arm pain was alleviated.

Treatment with Acupuncture and Related Therapies

A majority of the included 323 citations mentioned acupuncture therapies for managing CR symptoms (289 citations, 89.5%), while 20 recommended moxibustion therapy (6.2%), and 14 described a combination of acupuncture and moxibustion therapies (4.3%). The results suggest that acupuncture therapy might have been a popular management for CR symptoms in the past.

Seven citations mentioned the meridians for managing CR symptoms without specifying acupuncture points, including the Small Intestine meridian (4 citations), Bladder meridian (3 citations), Triple Energiser meridian (1 citation), Heart meridian (1 citation), Lung meridian (1 citation), and Large Intestine meridian (1 citation). For the vast majority of citations describing acupuncture points, the points were extracted and further analysed.

Most Frequent Acupuncture Points in Citations Possibly Related to Cervical Radiculopathy

A total of 98 acupuncture points were mentioned in the "possible CR" citations. The most frequently cited acupuncture points were mainly from three *yang* meridians of the hand, including the Large Intestine meridian (LI11 *Quchi* 曲池, LI15 *Jianyu* 肩髃, LI10 *Shousanli* 手三里, LI4 *Hegu* 合谷, LI12 *Zhouliao* 肘髎 and LI5 *Yangxi* 阳溪); the Triple Energiser meridian (TE5 *Waiguan* 外关, TE3 *Zhongzhu* 中渚,

Table 3.9.   Most Frequent Acupuncture Points in Possible Cervical Radiculopathy Citations

Acupuncture Point	No. of Citations (*n*)
LI11 *Quchi* 曲池	67
LI15 *Jianyu* 肩髃	44
GB21 *Jianjing* 肩井	43
LI10 *Shousanli* 手三里	31
LI4 *Hegu* 合谷	20
SI5 *Yanggu* 阳谷	20
SI4 *Wangu* 腕骨	19
SI2 *Qiangu* 前谷	17
TE5 *Waiguan* 外关	17
TE3 *Zhongzhu* 中渚	16
TE10 *Tianjing* 天井	15
TE11 *Tianzong* 天宗	15
SI3 *Houxi* 后溪	13
LU5 *Chize* 尺泽	12
LI12 *Zhouliao* 肘髎	12
TE4 *Yangchi* 阳池	10
TE2 *Yemen* 液门	10
TE14 *Jianliao* 肩髎	9
LI5 *Yangxi* 阳溪	9
TE6 *Zhigou* 支沟	9

TE10 *Tianjing* 天井, TE11 *Tianzong* 天宗, TE4 *Yangchi* 阳池, TE2 *Yemen* 液门 and TE6 *Zhigou* 支沟); and the Small Intestine meridian (SI5 *Yanggu* 阳谷, SI4 *Wangu* 腕骨, SI2 *Qiangu* 前谷 and SI3 *Houxi* 后溪) (Table 3.9). The three *yang* meridians run through the posterior aspect of the upper limbs from the hand crossing the shoulder to the head, which covers most CR-affected regions. Considering that the other most commonly cited points — GB21 *Jianjing* 肩井 and LU5 *Chize* 尺泽 — are also located on the upper limbs, this suggests the point selection principle was mainly based on nearby or local therapeutic effects of acupuncture points in past eras.

Most Frequent Acupuncture Points in Most Likely Cervical Radiculopathy Citations

There were 295 citations describing "pain" symptoms that were judged as "most likely CR" citations from the total pool. A total of 93 acupuncture points were obtained from the included citations. The most commonly recommended points are presented in Table 3.10. The majority of these points are also the most frequently cited acupuncture points in the total pool, showing that these were the most representative points for historically managing CR. The points SI14 *Jianwaishu* 肩外俞 (*n* = 9), located in the shoulder area, and HT3

Table 3.10.   Most Frequent Acupuncture Points in Most Likely Cervical Radiculopathy Citations

Acupuncture Point	No. of Citations (*n*)
LI11 *Quchi* 曲池	57
GB21 *Jianjing* 肩井	40
LI15 *Jianyu* 肩髃	37
LI10 *Shousanli* 手三里	26
SI5 *Yanggu* 阳谷	20
LI4 *Hegu* 合谷	16
SI2 *Qiangu* 前谷	16
SJ3 *Zhongzhu* 中渚	16
SI11 *Tianzhong* 天宗	15
SI4 *Wangu* 腕骨	15
SI3 *Houxi* 后溪	13
TE5 *Waiguan* 外关	13
TE10 *Tianjing* 天井	13
LI12 *Zhouliao* 肘髎	11
TE4 *Yangchi* 阳池	11
TE2 *Yemen* 液门	10
TE14 *Jianliao* 肩髎	10
SI14 *Jianwaishu* 肩外俞	9
HT3 *Shaohai* 少海	8
LU5 *Chize* 尺泽	8

Shaohai 少海 (*n* = 8), located in the elbow joint area, were found to be exclusively in the "most likely CR" citations pool. The point selection principle was consistent with the "possible CR" pool.

LI11 *Quchi* 曲池 was found to be the most frequently cited acupuncture point in classical literature. As early as the Jin 晋 dynasty (266–420 CE), the book *Zhen Jiu Jia Yi Jing* 针灸甲乙经 detailed that LI11 *Quchi* 曲池 could be used for managing shoulder, elbow and wrist pain, and restricted joint flexion, extension and mobility of the upper limbs (肩肘中痛, 难屈伸, 手不可举, 腕重急, 曲池主之). By stimulating this point, LI11 *Quchi* 曲池 has the functions to expel wind and heat, and relieve the obstruction of meridians and collateral vessels. In contemporary guidelines/textbooks, LI11 *Quchi* 曲池 is also recommended for CR with radial forearm numbness (see Chap. 2), which shows its importance in managing CR symptoms.

Discussion of Acupuncture for Cervical Radiculopathy

In the included classical literature evidence, acupuncture and/or moxibustion therapies were described in more than 300 citations in our evaluation. Most citations recommended acupuncture individually, which shows its importance and popularity in managing CR symptoms in past eras. The majority of the most frequently cited acupuncture points were from three *yang* meridians of the hand that covered most CR-affected areas from the neck and shoulder to the upper extremities. This indicates that the adjacent acupuncture point selection principle was commonly used historically, which is consistent with the point selection method in contemporary textbooks and guidelines (see Chap. 2). However, some major points located around the neck including the cervical EX-B2 *Jiaji* 颈夹脊 points, GV14 *Dazhui* 大椎 and BL10 *Tianzhu* 天柱, which are recommended in contemporary literature, were not commonly cited in classical books. One possible reason could be that cervical spinal diseases have been found to be the key pathologies that generate neck, shoulder and upper limb pain with advances in modern clinical Chinese medicine practice. The acupuncture point selection principle has been modified in light of this development.

Other Chinese Medicine Therapies

Other Chinese medicine therapies were found in nine citations, which were all judged as "most likely CR". Eight citations introduced *daoyin* 导引 exercise. Four citations were obtained from the Chao Yuan-Fang 巢元方 books *Zhu Bing Yuan Hou Lun* 诸病源候论 (610 CE) and *Cao Shi Bing Yuan Bu Yang Xuan Dao Fa* 巢氏病源补养宣导法 (610 CE), published before the Tang dynasty. The others were found in books published in the Ming dynasty (1369–1644 CE, 3 citations) and Qing dynasty (1645–1911 CE, 2 citations).

In the *Zhu Bing Yuan Hou Lun* 诸病源候论, the author mentioned a *qigong*-style *daoyin* 导引 exercise for managing thigh, leg and arm pain: "Ask the patient to lie down on his back and make him hold his breath until he feels abdominal pain, then push the abdominal pain with his mind and meditation towards the affected limb area. As the patient's mind pushes the *qi* to the painful area, he will feel heat throughout his body and the pain can be relieved (治股, 胫, 手臂痛法: 屈一胫, 臂中所痛者, 正偃卧, 口鼻闭气, 腹痛, 以意推之, 想气往至痛上, 俱热即愈)".

The exercise style *daoyin* was introduced in several citations. Hu Wen-Huan 胡文焕 in his book *Yang Sheng Dao Yin Fa* 养生导引法 (1368 CE) described that "raising the head and shoulder, shaking the head and breathing exercises could be used for managing spinal and neck pain 脊椎及颈项痛, 可采用仰面抬肩, 左右摇头的动作和吐纳法". In the book *Shou Shi Chuan Zhen* 寿世传真 (1771 CE), the author, Xu Wen-Bi 徐文弼, recommended another exercise to manage shoulder pain: "Ask the patient to cross his hands at the neck, then raise his head, push his hands towards his neck and lean his neck towards his hands at the same time (一两手相叉抱项后, 面仰视, 使手与项争力)".

Massage therapy was mentioned in one citation, obtained from the book *Shi Shi Mi Lu* 石室秘录 (1687 CE). The author wrote that "massage therapy was beneficial for the flowing of *qi* and Blood, and treating phlegm disease (法当以人手为之按摩, 则气血流通, 痰病易愈). The practitioner could relieve the patient's hand and foot pain by compressing movement (执其两手, 捻之者千下而后已, 左右手各如是, 一日之间, 而手足之疼痛可已)".

Classical Literature in Perspective

According to classical Chinese medicine literature, CR was not considered a specific clinical condition. The main symptoms of CR were mentioned under other disease names or symptoms such as *Bi* (1) disease 痹证, *bi* (2) *tong* 臂痛 (arm pain), and *jian tong* 肩痛 (shoulder pain). A comprehensive search using relevant disease names and symptoms in classical terminology was conducted in the ZHYD — 23,677 hits (instances) were obtained. In order to select the citations that were possible or most likely referring to CR, we applied rigorous selection criteria of:

- Citations that described at least two location terms and any representative symptom terms were judged as "possible CR" citations.
- Citations that contained at least two location terms and pain symptoms (*teng* 疼 or *tong* 痛) were determined as "most likely CR" citations.

As a result, a total of 684 citations met the inclusion criteria and were considered "possible CR", and 627 of these 684 were further judged as "most likely CR" citations because they described the most representative "pain" symptom in their texts. Due to the similar number of citations included in these two pools, the treatments extracted from the citations of the two pools are very similar.

Fifty-seven citations mentioned at least two location terms and any representative symptom terms without any pain symptoms. These citations all mentioned numbness as the main symptom. The CHM treatments involved in these citations target tonifying *qi* and eliminating phlegm, for example, *Bu zhong yi qi tang* 补中益气汤 and *Fu ling wan* 茯苓丸. The acupuncture points introduced by these citations were similar to those included in the "most likely CRS" citations.

The Chinese medicine aetiology of CR was also recorded in some citations that did not introduce any treatment. As a summary of the descriptions of aetiology, the main aetiology and pathogenesis of this condition were: invasion of wind, cold and dampness pathological factors, phlegm, and traumatic injury.

In terms of the relevant CHM treatment, our evaluation found that the majority of CHM treatments were oral CHM formulae. The most frequently used ones were: *Fu ling wan/Zhi mi fu ling wan/Zhi mi wan* 茯苓丸/指迷茯苓丸/指迷丸, *Juan bi tang/Juan bi tang jia jian* 蠲痹汤/蠲痹汤加减, *Er chen tang/Er chen tang jia jian* 二陈汤/二陈汤加减, *Dao tan tang/Dao tan tang jia jian* 导痰汤/导痰汤加减, *Kong xian dan/Kong xian dan jia jian* 控涎丹/控涎丹加减, *Wu ji san/Wu ji san jia jian* 五积散/五积散加减, *Wu yao shun qi san/Wu yao shun qi san jia jian* 乌药顺气散/乌药顺气散加减, *Shu jing tang* 舒筋汤, *Gun tan wan* 滚痰丸 and *Qiang huo sheng shi tang* 羌活胜湿汤. Based on these common formulae included in the "most likely CR" pool, it could be seen that the treatment principles are eliminating phlegm, wind, cold and dampness pathological factors. The most frequently used herbs are: *Gan cao* 甘草, *fu ling* 茯苓, *ban xia* 半夏, *sheng jiang/gan jiang* 生姜/干姜, *dang gui* 当归, *qiang huo* 羌活, *shao yao/chi shao/bai shao* 芍药/赤芍/白芍, *zhi ke* 枳壳, *chen pi* 陈皮 and *fang feng* 防风. These herbs also serve the treatment principle of eliminating phlegm and wind, cold and dampness pathological factors.

It is worth mentioning that Blood-moving herbs did not seem to be the most frequently used ones, reflecting that Blood stasis may not have played an important role in the aetiology of CR in the included citations. As stated above, the Ming and Qing dynasties (1368–1911 CE) produced the highest numbers of relevant books and included citations. In grouping the included citations by dynasty, it was found that practitioners before the Ming dynasty commonly treated this condition from the point of view of *qi* stagnation with Blood stasis 气血凝滞, as well as wind, cold and dampness 风寒湿邪. During the Ming and Qing dynasties, phlegm and dampness 痰湿 dominated the analysis of the aetiology of CR. During the Minguo period (1911–1949 CE), medical books recorded many detailed case reports stating that wind, cold and dampness 风寒湿邪 and *qi* stagnation with Blood stasis 气滞血瘀 were again the common etiology of CR, while phlegm and dampness 痰湿 became unpopular. In fact, Chinese medicine practice in China during the Minguo period was largely influenced by Western medicine, as shown in the book *Yi Lin Gai*

Cuo 医林改错 (1830 CE). The switch in CR aetiology reflects the development and evolution of Chinese medicine in history. Since this research was based on frequency analysis, it is not surprising that CHM formulae and herbs targeting resolving phlegm and dampness 痰湿 were shown as the most popular ones, since most of the citations were found in books published during the Ming and Qing dynasties. Such results should be interpreted with caution.

Topically used CHM was rarely seen in the pool of "most likely CR" citations. Only two citations listed details for using CHM topically, both introducing CHM hot packs.

As for acupuncture treatment, the frequently used acupuncture points recorded in the "most likely CR" citations were all located on the shoulder and arm, with LI11 *Quchi* 曲池 being the most frequently used one. These results indicate that the acupuncture treatments recorded in classical literature mainly focused on the local region of symptoms. Acupuncture therapy often applies Chinese medicine syndrome differentiation based on meridians, rather than the *zang* and *fu* theories. The symptoms of CR mainly appear on the upper extremities, which are the location of three hand *Yang* meridians and three hand *Yin* meridians. Therefore, the acupuncture points of these meridians were frequently selected to be used for relieving CR symptoms.

Daoyin 导引 exercise was identified in the classical literature, but no citations on *tuina* 推拿 therapy have been found.

References

1. Needham J, Lu G, Sivin N. (2000) *Science and Civilisation in China. Vol. 5, Part VI: Medicine.* Cambridge University Press, Cambridge.
2. 黄桂成. (2018) 中医骨伤科学. 中国中医药出版社, 北京.
3. May, BH, Lu Y, Lu C, *et al.* (2013) Systematic assessment of the representativeness of published collections of the traditional literature on Chinese medicine. *J Altern Complement Med* **19**(5): 403–409.
4. May BH, Lu C, Xue CC. (2012) Collections of traditional Chinese medical literature as resources for systematic searches. *J Altern Complement Med* **18**(12): 1101–1107.

5. 李新建. (2006) 筋伤内伤与骨病临床诊治. 科学技术文献出版社, 北京.

6. 孙树椿. (2011) 今日中医骨伤科. 人民卫生出版社, 北京.

7. 曾凡钢. (2018) 针刺联合冲击波对老年性神经根型颈椎病的临床疗效观察 (Thesis). 福建中医药大学.

8. 陈广林. (2018) 低温等离子联合中药治疗神经根型颈椎病的疗效观察及其机制的初步研究 (Thesis). 南京中医药大学.

9. 赖梦婷. (2018) 巨刺法配合颈椎牵引治疗神经根型颈椎病急性期的临床疗效观察 (Thesis). 福建中医药大学.

10. 李留鹏. (2018) 针刺联合TDP, 拔罐配合穴位磁疗对颈型颈椎病的临床疗效观察 (Thesis). 福建中医药大学.

11. 李妮娜. (2018) 基于"温阳调气法"针灸治疗风寒阻络证神经根型颈椎病的临床观察 (Thesis). 广西中医药大学.

12. 吕更宽. (2017) 艾灸治疗神经根型颈椎病的疗效观察及红外温度变化 (Thesis). 福建中医药大学.

13. 王崑萌. (2018) 针刺对颈椎病家兔作用机理的研究 (Thesis). 福建中医药大学.

14. 徐铭阳. (2018) 针刀治疗神经根型颈椎病的临床疗效观察 (Thesis). 湖北中医药大学.

15. 杨金贵. (2018) 颈椎通络胶囊治疗神经根型颈椎病（寒瘀阻络证）的临床疗效观察 (Thesis). 黑龙江中医药大学.

16. 张倩倩. (2017) 不同针刺深度对神经根型颈椎病肌电图改变的对比观察 (Thesis). 山东中医药大学.

17. 周仲瑛. (2003) 中医内科学. 中国中医药出版社, 北京.

18. 国家中医药管理局'十一五'重点专科协作组. (2017) 项痹病(神经根型颈椎病)诊疗方案.

19. Rebera A. (2019) *Poisons Standard February 2019*. Available from: www.legislation.gov.au/Details/F2019L00032.

4

Methods for Evaluating Clinical Evidence

OVERVIEW

This chapter describes the methods used to identify and evaluate a range of Chinese medicine interventions for cervical radiculopathy in clinical studies. Studies identified through a comprehensive search have been assessed against eligibility criteria. A review of the methodological quality of the studies has been undertaken using standardised methods. Results from the included studies have been evaluated to provide an estimate of the effects of a range of Chinese medicine therapies.

Introduction

The use of Chinese medicine for cervical radiculopathy (CR) has been well described in contemporary literature (see Chapter 2) and classical Chinese medicine (see Chapter 3). The evidence for Chinese medicine therapies from modern literature will be presented in subsequent chapters. This chapter describes the methods used to evaluate clinical studies. Studies have been evaluated following the methods of the *Cochrane Handbook of Systematic Reviews*.[1] Interventions have been categorised as follows:

- Chinese herbal medicine (CHM) (Chapter 5)
- Acupuncture and related therapies (Chapter 7)
- Other CM therapies (Chapter 8)
- Chinese medicine combination therapies (Chapter 9).

Table 4.1.   Chinese Medicine Interventions Included in Clinical Evidence Evaluation

Category	Intervention
Chinese herbal medicine (Chapter 5)	Oral Chinese herbal medicine and topical Chinese herbal medicine.
Acupuncture and related therapies (Chapter 7)	Acupuncture, electroacupuncture, ear acupuncture, moxibustion, warm needling and other types of acupuncture.
Other Chinese medicine therapies (Chapter 8)	*Tuina* 推拿 therapy and *daoyin* 导引 therapy.
Chinese medicine combination therapy (Chapter 9)	Chinese medicine combination therapy is defined as two or more Chinese medicine interventions from different categories administered together, e.g., Chinese herbal medicine plus acupuncture and Chinese herbal medicine plus ear acupressure.

References to clinical trials were obtained and assessed by an expert group. Randomised controlled trials (RCTs), non-randomised controlled clinical trials (CCTs) and non-controlled studies were evaluated in detail. CCTs were evaluated using the same approach as for RCTs and are described separately. Evidence from non-controlled studies is more difficult to evaluate, therefore an approach was taken to describe the characteristics of the study, details of the intervention and any adverse events. References to included studies are indicated by a letter followed by a number. Studies of CHM are indicated by "H", e.g., H1; studies of acupuncture-related therapies are indicated by "A", e.g., A1; studies of other Chinese medicine therapies are indicated by "O", e.g., O1; and studies of Chinese medicine combination therapy (see Table 4.1) are indicated by "C", e.g., C1.

Search Strategy

Evidence was searched for in English- and Chinese-language databases and the methods followed the *Cochrane Handbook of Systematic Reviews.*[1] English-language databases included PubMed, the Excerpta Medica Database (Embase), Cumulative Index of

Nursing and Allied Health Literature (CINAHL), and the Cochrane Central Register of Controlled Trials (CENTRAL), including the Cochrane Library, and Allied and Complementary Medicine Database (AMED). Chinese-language databases included China BioMedical Literature (CBM), China National Knowledge Infrastructure (CNKI), Chongqing VIP (CQVIP), and Wanfang. Databases were searched from inception to January 2019. No restrictions were applied. Search terms were mapped to controlled vocabulary (where applicable), in addition to being searched as keywords.

To conduct a comprehensive search of the literature, searches were run according to the study design (reviews, controlled trials and non-controlled studies). This was done for each of the three intervention types (CHM, acupuncture and related therapies, and other Chinese medicine therapies) resulting in nine searches in each of the nine databases:

1. CHM — reviews;
2. CHM — controlled trials (randomised and non-randomised);
3. CHM — non-controlled studies;
4. Acupuncture and related therapies — reviews;
5. Acupuncture and related therapies — controlled trials (randomised and non-randomised);
6. Acupuncture and related therapies — non-controlled studies;
7. Other Chinese medicine therapies — reviews;
8. Other Chinese medicine therapies — controlled trials (randomised and non-randomised); and
9. Other Chinese medicine therapies — non-controlled studies.

Studies of Chinese medicine combination therapy were identified through the above searches. In addition to electronic databases, the reference lists of systematic reviews and included studies were searched for additional publications. Clinical trial registries were searched to identify ongoing or completed clinical trials, and where required, trial investigators were contacted to obtain data. The searched trial registries included the Australian New Zealand Clinical Trial Registry (ANZCTR), Chinese Clinical Trial Registry (ChiCTR), European Union Clinical Trials

Register (EU-CTR), and the United States of America National Institutes of Health register (ClinicalTrials.gov).

Inclusion Criteria

- Participants: Patients who were diagnosed with CR following the diagnostic criteria defined in clinical guidelines, e.g., an evidence-based clinical guideline for the diagnosis and treatment of cervical radiculopathy from degenerative disorders,[2] and national clinical guidelines for non-surgical treatment of patients with recent onset neck pain or cervical radiculopathy;[3]
- Interventions: CHM, acupuncture and related therapies, or other Chinese medicine therapies, alone or in combination with pharmacotherapy/routine care (Table 4.1), and studies combining Chinese medicine therapies with pharmacotherapy/routine care required the use of the same pharmacotherapy/routine care in both the intervention and comparator groups;
- Comparators: Placebo, no treatment, pharmacotherapies or other routine care therapies that are recommended in international clinical practice guidelines; and
- Outcome measures: Studies reported at least one of the pre-specified outcome measures (Table 4.2).

Table 4.2.   Pre-Specified Outcomes

Outcome Categories	Outcome Measures	Scoring
Pain	1. Visual Analogue Scale (VAS)	0 to 10 or 0 to 100, lower is better
	2. Numeric Rating Scale (NRS)	0 to 10 or 0 to 100, lower is better
	3. McGill Pain Questionnaire (MPQ)	0 to 78, lower is better
	4. Northwick Park Neck Pain Questionnaire	0% to 100%, lower is better

Table 4.2.   (*Continued*)

Outcome Categories	Outcome Measures	Scoring
Cervical Spondylosis specific outcome measures	Neck Disability Index (NDI)	0% to 100%, lower is better
	Scoring System for Cervical Radiculopathy (SSCR)	0 to 20, higher is better
	Assessment Scale for Cervical Spondylosis (ASCS)	0 to 29, higher is better
	Outcome Assessment System in the Treatment of Cervical Radiculopathy (OASTCR)	0 to 35, lower is better
	Clinical Assessment Scale for Cervical Spondylosis (CASCS)	0 to 100, higher is better
Effective rate	Effective rate	0% to 100%, higher is better
Patient reported quality of life outcome	Short Form (36) Health Survey (SF-36)	0 to 100, higher is better
Adverse events	Number and type of adverse events	

Exclusion Criteria

- Studies recruited participants not limited to CR, e.g., participants were diagnosed with other types of cervical spondylosis or a combination of different types of cervical spondylosis;
- Studies that used Chinese medicine therapies as the comparator or used different routine therapies between the intervention and control groups;
- Studies that did not report data on the pre-defined outcomes (Table 4.2); and
- Duplicated studies that reported the same results; those published later were excluded.

Outcomes

In an evidence-based clinical practice guideline developed by the North American Spine Society (NASS) in 2010, it was stated that the

Neck Disability Index (NDI), Short Form (36) Health Survey (SF-36), 12-Item Short Form Survey (SF-12) and pain Visual Analogue Scale (VAS) are recommended outcome measures for assessing the treatment of cervical radiculopathy from degenerative disorders (Grade of recommendation: A). Other outcome measures with a level B Grade of recommendation are: The Modified Prolo, Patient Specific Functional Scale (PSFS), Health Status Questionnaire, Sickness Impact Profile, Modified Million Index, McGill Pain Questionnaire (MPQ) and Modified Oswestry Disability Index.[2] In the Danish national clinical guideline published in 2017, it is suggested that the primary outcomes of CR are pain and pain-related activity limitations.[3] For these outcomes, the absolute differences between the intervention and control groups on generally accepted and validated instruments such as the pain VAS, numeric rating scale (NRS) or NDI should be selected.[3]

In addition, our comprehensive evaluation found that there was a few other outcome measures commonly reported in clinical research conducted in China. In order to comprehensively evaluate the clinical evidence, both those outcome measures recommended by international clinical guidelines and those commonly used in clinical studies were considered (Table 4.2). Detailed contents and methods of these outcome measures are summarised next.

Pain Visual Analogue Scale

The VAS is a 10 cm line, oriented vertically or horizontally, with one end representing "no pain" and the other end representing "pain as bad as it can be". The patient is asked to mark a place on the line corresponding to the current pain intensity. The VAS is the most frequently used pain measure because it is simple to use and has good psychometric properties.[4–10]

Numeric Rating Scale

The NRS, designed by Budzynski and Melzack, is another widely used measurement instrument to verify pain intensity. The NRS is a verbal or written determination of a pain level on a scale from 0 to 10, in which 0 represents no pain and 10 represents excruciating pain. Sternbach has expanded the NRS to a rating from 0 to 100, and the patient is asked to describe current or average pain intensity as a percentage out of 100.[3]

When comparing the VAS with the NRS, some investigators have stated that the NRS is not as sensitive to patients' ability to express distress, and therefore they recommend using the VAS because it is better suited to parametric analysis and because it provides a continuous score.[11]

McGill Pain Questionnaire

The MPQ is a self-reporting measure of pain used for patients with a number of diagnoses.[12] It was the first tool (developed in 1975) to offer a multidimensional assessment of pain, which included an assessment of severity or intensity, emotional impact and significance to the pain sufferer.[13]

The MPQ is comprised of 78 words, of which respondents choose those that best describe their experience of pain. It consists of 20 sets of verbal descriptors, ordered in intensity from lowest to highest:

- Dimension 1: Pain descriptors (set 1 to 10);
- Dimension 2: Affective components of pain (set 11 to 15);
- Dimension 3: Evaluation of pain (set 16); and
- Dimension 4: Miscellaneous (set 17 to 20).

Patients are required to select the words that describe their pain. Qualitative differences in pain may be reflected in the word choices from respondents. The quantitative data is summed to form the Pain Rating Index (PRI), which includes PRI-Total (PRI-T; score 0–78), PRI-Sensory (PRI-S; score 0–42), PRI-Affective (PRI-A; score 0–14), PRI-Evaluative (PRI-E; score 0–5), and PRI-Miscellaneous (PRI-M; score 0–17).[14] Higher scores indicate more severe pain.[12,15]

Considering that the standard MPQ takes a long time to administer, a short form of the MPQ (SF-MPQ) was developed in 1987.[16] The main component of the SF-MPQ consists of 15 descriptors (11 sensory; 4 affective), which are rated on an intensity scale of 0 = none, 1 = mild, 2 = moderate and 3 = severe. Three pain scores are derived from the sum of the intensity rank values of the words chosen for the sensory, affective and total descriptors. The SF-MPQ also includes the Present Pain Intensity (PPI) index of the standard MPQ and a VAS. The MPQ and its later derivative, the SF-MPQ, have been used widely in both experimental and clinical pain studies.[13]

Northwick Park Neck Pain Questionnaire

The Northwick Park Neck Pain Questionnaire (NPQ) measures neck pain and consequent patient disabilities. It is easy to complete, simple to score and provides an objective measure to evaluate outcome and to monitor symptoms in patients with acute or chronic neck pain over time.[17]

The questionnaire is divided into nine sections: (1) Neck pain intensity, (2) Neck pain and sleeping, (3) Pins and needles or numbness in the arms at night, (4) Duration of symptoms, (5) Carrying, (6) Reading and watching television, (7) Working and/or housework, (8) Social activities and (9) Driving. At the end there is a tenth question that aims to compare the current state to the state when the questionnaire was last completed.[17] Each parameter is divided into five answer possibilities with points from 0 (meaning no pain) to 4 (the worst pain). Patients are required to fill in the questions. The neck pain score is the sum of the points scored for the first nine questions. The interpretation is done by the clinicians. The minimum score is 0. The maximum score is 36 if all nine questions are answered and 32 if only the first eight questions are answered. The percentage ranges from 0% to 100%. The higher the percentage, the greater the disability and the pain.[17]

Neck Disability Index

The NDI determines the extent of disability and is designed to measure activity limitations due to neck pain and disability. It is the most frequently used functional outcome tool for cervical-related disabilities.[18] The NDI is a 10-item questionnaire designed to assess neck pain and disability.[19] This scale is based on the Oswestry Index, which is a 10-item measure designed to assess pain-related limitations in activities of daily living.[20] The NDI is scored using a percentage of the maximal pain and disability score. The items are organised by type of activity and followed by six different assertions expressing progressive levels of functional capability.

The Short Form (36) Health Survey

The SF-36 is a 36-item, patient-reported survey of patient health. The SF-36 is a measure of health status, which is commonly used in health economics as a variable in the quality-adjusted life year cal-culation to determine the cost-effectiveness of a health treatment. The SF-36 consists of eight scaled scores, which are the weighted sums of the questions in their section. The eight sections are:

- Vitality;
- Physical functioning;
- Bodily pain;
- General health perceptions;
- Physical role functioning;
- Emotional role functioning;
- Social role functioning; and
- Mental health.

Each scale is directly transformed into a 0–100 scale on the assumption that each question carries equal weight. The lower the score the greater the disability, while the higher the score the lesser the disability.[21] Some outcome measures are commonly used in clinical research in China, as described next.

Effective Rate

The effective rate is an outcome measure that is commonly used in clinical trials conducted in China. The effective rate has been recommended by several national clinical guidelines in China for CR including:

- In the *Standards for Diagnosis and Treatment Effects Evaluation in Chinese Medicine* (1994 version) (中医病症诊断疗效标准 1994 版本),[22] the treatment effects were defined with three levels: Clinical cured, effective and ineffective;
- In *Principle for Clinical Research on New Chinese Herbal Medicine Drugs* (2002 version) (中药新药临床研究指导原则试行 2002 版本),[23] they were defined with four levels: Clinical cured, significantly effective, effective and ineffective; and
- In the *Clinical Guideline for Chinese Medicine Clinical Diagnosis and Treatment of 95 Diseases* (2001 version) (22 个专业 95 个病种中医诊疗方案 2001 版本),[24] a scoring system was introduced for calculating the effectiveness. Based on a reduction of symptom scores, the treatment effects were defined as four levels: Clinical cured, significantly effective, effective and ineffective (reduction >90%, 70–90%, 30–70% and ≤30%, respectively).

Most of the clinical studies conducted in China applied the effective rate as a common outcome measure following different definitions of "clinical cured" or "effective". In this monograph, we merged the results "clinical cured", "significantly effective" and "effective" into "effective", and therefore the results were grouped as "effective" and "ineffective" for meta-analysis.

Scoring System for Cervical Radiculopathy

The Scoring System for Cervical Radiculopathy (SSCR) was proposed by Tanaka *et al.* in 1993 to evaluate pain, disability and neurological status.[25] This scoring system consists of 20 items grouped in the following four categories: (1) Subjective symptoms, (2) Ability to work, (3) Finger function and (4) Objective signs. Three symptoms are included in the "Subjective symptoms" category: Neck symptoms, arm symptoms and finger symptoms. Four items are included in the "Objective signs" category: Spurling's test, sensory function, motor function and deep tendon reflex. Scores are given to each item with the total score ranging from −2 to 20; lower scores indicate more severe symptoms and disability.[25]

This scoring system was translated into Chinese in 1996,[26] since then it has been frequently used in clinical studies conducted in China. The translated version of this outcome measure was named after the first author and is commonly known as 田中靖久颈椎病症状量表 in China. In this monograph, we present its results under the original name of this scoring system, which is the SSCR.

Assessment Scale for Cervical Spondylosis

The Assessment Scale for Cervical Spondylosis (ASCS) was developed by Wang *et al.*[27] This scale consists of three sections:

- Section 1: Total score of 29 points; lower scores indicate more severe symptoms, including:
  - Clinical symptoms;
  - Clinical examination including six examinations;
  - Quality-of-life questions; and
  - Patients' satisfaction with treatment;
- Section 2: Pain VAS; and
- Section 3: Objective examinations including X-ray, computed tomography (CT) or magnetic resonance imaging (MRI) scans.

This scale is considered a comprehensive evaluation since it also involves objective examinations. However, the reliability and validity of this scale have not been confirmed.

Outcome Assessment System in the Treatment of Cervical Radiculopathy

The Outcome Assessment System in the Treatment of Cervical Radiculopathy (OASTCR) was developed by Zhu *et al.*[28] This scale combines the SSCR and pain evaluation using the NRS, and contains nine items with a total score of 35, where higher scores indicate a more severe condition. The nine items cover clinical symptoms (2 questions) and objective evaluations (7 questions). Compared with the SSCR, this scale is considered more objective for evaluating the treatment effects for CR because it adds three clinical examinations: Cervical pressing pain, cervical range of motion and the Brachial plexus nerve traction test.

Clinical Assessment Scale for Cervical Spondylosis

The Clinical Assessment Scale for Cervical Spondylosis (CASCS) is an outcome measure assessing the symptoms, clinical signs and function status of all types of cervical spondylosis patients.[29] This scale was developed by Zhang *et al.*, and the reliability, validity and sensitivity of this scale have been shown by previous studies.

This scale contains 13 items belonging to three domains: Subjective symptoms, life and work ability, and clinical signs. The total score is 100 points, of which 73 points are based on clinical examination and clinical signs. Only 18 points are based on patients' symptoms and 9 points on patients' life and work ability. In fact, in CR patients, the treatment goal should be to target the severity of subjective symptoms rather than clinical examination results. In addition, completing all the assessments included in this scale is quite time-consuming.

Risk-of-Bias Assessment

The risk of bias was assessed for RCTs using the Cochrane Collaboration tool.[1] In clinical trials, bias can be categorised as selection bias, performance bias, detection bias, attrition bias and reporting bias. Each domain is assessed to determine whether the bias is of a "low", "high" or "unclear" risk. "Low" risk of bias indicates that bias is unlikely, a "high" risk indicates plausible bias that seriously weakens confidence in the results, and an "unclear" bias indicates a lack of information or uncertainty over potential bias and raises some doubt about the results. Risk-of-bias assessments were verified by two people, and any disagreement was resolved by discussion or consultation with a third person.

Risk of bias is categorised using the following six domains:

- **Sequence generation**: The method used to generate the allocation sequence is given in sufficient detail to allow an assessment of whether it should produce comparable groups. A "low" risk of bias refers to a random number table or computer random generator. A "high" risk of bias includes studies that describe a non-random sequence generation such as odd or even dates of birth or dates of admission.
- **Allocation concealment**: The method used to conceal the allocation sequence is given in enough detail to determine whether intervention allocations could have been foreseen before or during enrolment. A "low" risk of bias includes central randomisation or sealed envelopes and a "high" risk of bias includes open random sequences or dates of birth, etc.
- **Blinding of participants and personnel**: Measures used to describe whether the study participants and personnel were blind to the intervention received. In addition, information relating to whether the blinding was effective is also assessed. Studies that ensured the blinding of participants and personnel are at "low" risk of bias. If a study was not blind or incompletely blind, it is at a "high" risk of bias.
- **Blinding of outcome assessors**: Measures used to describe whether the outcome assessors were blind to the knowledge of which intervention a participant received. In addition, information relating to whether the blinding was effective is also assessed. Studies that ensured blinding of outcome assessors are at "low" risk of bias. If a study was not blind or incompletely blind, it is at a "high" risk of bias.
- **Incomplete outcome data**: Completeness of outcome data for each main outcome, including dropouts, exclusions from the analysis with numbers missing in each group and reasons for

dropouts and exclusions. Studies with "low" risk of bias included all outcome data, or if there was missing data, it was unlikely to relate to the true outcome or was balanced between groups. Studies at "high" risk of bias have unexplained missing data.

- **Selective reporting**: The study protocol is available, and the pre-specified outcomes are included in the report. Studies with a published protocol and which include all pre-specified outcomes in their report are at a "low" risk of bias. Studies at a "high" risk of bias did not include all pre-specified outcomes, or the outcome data was reported incompletely.

Statistical Analyses

The frequency of Chinese medicine syndromes and the CHM formulae, herbs and acupuncture points reported in included studies are presented using descriptive statistics. Chinese medicine syndromes reported in two or more studies are also presented. The 10 most frequently reported CHM formulae and 20 most frequently reported herbs are presented where used in at least two studies, although for CHM formulae this was not always possible. The top 10 acupuncture points used in two or more studies are presented, or as available. Where data was limited, reports of single Chinese medicine syndromes or acupuncture points are provided as a guide for the reader.

Definitions of statistical tests and results are described in the Glossary. Dichotomous data is reported as the risk ratio (RR) with a 95% confidence interval (CI), and continuous data is reported as the mean difference (MD) or standard mean difference (SMD) with a 95% CI. For dichotomous data, when the RR is greater than one and the upper and lower values of the 95% CI are both greater than one, this indicates we can be 95% certain that there is a difference between the groups and that the true effect lies within these CIs. The same is true for values less than one. In such cases, we say there is a "significant difference" between the groups. For continuous data, when the MD is greater than zero and both the upper and lower values of the 95% CI are greater than zero, we say there is a "significant difference" between the groups. The same is true on the negative side of the scale.[1]

For all analyses, RR, MD or SMD, together with a 95% CI, are reported, together with a formal test for heterogeneity using the I^2 statistic. An I^2 score greater than 50% is considered to indicate substantial heterogeneity.[1] Sensitivity analyses were undertaken to explore potential sources of heterogeneity, based on a "low" risk of bias for one of the risk-of-bias domains — sequence generation. Where possible and appropriate, planned subgroup analyses included the severity of the disease, duration of treatment, Chinese medicine formulae, and comparator types. An available case analysis with a random effects model was used in all analyses. The random effects model was used to take into account the clinical heterogeneity likely to be encountered within and between included studies, and the variation in treatment effects between included studies.

Assessment Using Grading of Recommendations Assessment, Development and Evaluation

The Grading of Recommendations Assessment, Development and Evaluation (GRADE) approach was used.[30] The GRADE approach summarises and rates the strength and quality (certainty) of evidence in systematic reviews using a structured process for presenting evidence summaries. The results are presented in summary of findings tables. The results provide an important overview of CR outcomes.

A panel of experts was established to evaluate the certainty of evidence. The panel included the systematic review team, Chinese medicine practitioners, integrative medicine experts, research methodologists, and conventional medicine physicians. The experts were asked to rate the clinical importance of key interventions from CHM, acupuncture therapies and other Chinese medicine therapies, as well as comparators and outcomes. Results were collated and based on the rating scores, and via subsequent discussion, a consensus on the content for the summary of findings tables was achieved.

The certainty of evidence for each outcome was rated according to five factors outlined in the GRADE approach. The certainty of evidence may be rated based on:

- Limitations in study design (risk of bias);
- Inconsistency of results (unexplained heterogeneity);
- Indirectness of evidence (interventions, populations and outcomes important to the patients with the condition);
- Imprecision (uncertainty about the results); and
- Publication bias (selective publication of studies).

These five factors are additive and a reduction in one or more factors will reduce the certainty of the evidence for that outcome. The GRADE approach also includes methods for assessing observational studies. GRADE summaries in this monograph only include RCTs.

Treatment recommendations can also be assessed using the GRADE approach, but due to the diverse nature of Chinese medicine practice, treatment recommendations are not included with the summary of findings. Therefore, the reader should interpret the evidence with reference to the local practice environment. It should also be noted that the GRADE approach requires judgements about the strength and certainty of evidence and some subjective assessment. However, the experience of the panel members suggests these judgements are reliable and transparent representations of the certainty of evidence. The GRADE levels of evidence are grouped into four categories:

1) "High" certainty: We are very confident that the true effect lies close to the estimate of the effect;
2) "Moderate" certainty: We are moderately confident in the effect estimate and the true effect is likely to be close to the estimate of the effect, but there is a possibility that it is substantially different;
3) "Low" certainty: Our confidence in the effect estimate is limited and the true effect may be substantially different from the estimate of the effect; and

4) "Very low" certainty: We have very little confidence in the effect estimate and the true effect is likely to be substantially different from the estimate of effect.

References

1. Higgins J, Green S. (eds.) (2011) *Cochrane Handbook for Systematic Reviews of Interventions Version 5.1.0* (Cochrane Collaboration). Retrieved from: www.cochrane-handbook.org.
2. Bono CM, Ghiselli G, Gilbert TJ, *et al.* (2011) An evidence-based clinical guideline for the diagnosis and treatment of cervical radiculopathy from degenerative disorders. *Spine J* **11**(1): 64–72.
3. Kjaer P, Kongsted A, Hartvigsen J, *et al.* (2017) National clinical guidelines for non-surgical treatment of patients with recent onset neck pain or cervical radiculopathy. *Eur Spine J* **26**(9): 2242–2257.
4. Ylinen J, Salo P, Nykanen M, *et al.* (2004) Decreased isometric neck muscle strength in women with chronic neck pain and the repeatability of neck strength measurements. *Arch Phys Med Rehabil* **85**(8): 1303–1308.
5. Price DD, McGrath PA, Rafii A, Buckingham B. (1983) The validation of visual analogue scales as ratio scale measures for chronic and experimental pain. *Pain* **17**(1): 45–56.
6. Bijur PE, Silver W, Gallagher EJ. (2001) Reliability of the visual analogue scale for measurement of acute pain. *Acad Emerg Med* **8**(12): 1153–1157.
7. Gonzalez T, Balsa A, Sainz DM, *et al.* (2001) Spanish version of the Northwick Park Neck Pain Questionnaire: Reliability and validity. *Clin Exp Rheumatol* **19**(1): 41–46.
8. Wainner RS, Fritz JM, Boninger M, *et al.* (2003) Reliability and diagnostic accuracy of the clinical examination and patient self-report measures for cervical radiculopathy. *Spine* **28**(1): 52–62.
9. Bicer A, Yazici A, Camdeviren H, Erdogan C. (2004) Assessment of pain and disability in patients with chronic neck pain: Reliability and construct validity of the Turkish version of the neck pain and disability scale. *Disabil Rehabil* **26**(16): 959–962.
10. Wlodyka-Demaille S, Poiraudeau S, Catanzariti JF, *et al.* (2004) The ability to change of three questionnaires for neck pain. *Spine* **71**(4): 317–326.

11. Good M, Stiller C, Zauszniewski JA, *et al.* (2001) Sensation and distress of pain scales: Reliability, validity, and sensitivity. *J Nurs Meas* **9**(3): 219–238.

12. Melzack R. (1975) The McGill Pain Questionnaire: Major properties and scoring methods. *Pain* **1**(3): 277–299.

13. Main CJ. (2016) Pain assessment in context: A state of the science review of the McGill Pain Questionnaire 40 years on. *Pain* **157**(7): 1387–1399.

14. Katz J, Melzack R. (1999) Pain control in the perioperative period: Measurement of pain. *Surg Clin North Am* **79**(2): 231–252.

15. Ngamkham S, Vincent C, Finnegan L, *et al.* (2012) The McGill Pain Questionnaire as a multidimensional measure in people with cancer: An integrative review. *Pain Manag Nurs* **13**(1): 27–51.

16. Melzack R. (1987) The short-form McGill Pain Questionnaire. *Pain* **30**(2): 191–197.

17. Vernon H, Mior S. (1994) The Northwick Park Neck Pain Questionnaire, devised to measure neck pain and disability. *Br J Rheumatol* **33**(12): 1203–1204.

18. Pietrobon R, Coeytaux RR, Carey TS, Richardson WJ, DeVellis RF. (2002) Standard scales for measurement of functional outcome for cervical pain or dysfunction: A systematic review. *Spine* **27**(5): 515–522.

19. Vernon H, Mior S. (1991) The Neck Disability Index: A study of reliability and validity. *J Manipulative Physiol Ther* **14**(7): 409–415.

20. Fairbank JC, Couper J, Davies JB, O'Brien JP. (1980) The Oswestry Low Back Pain Disability Questionnaire. *Physiotherapy* **66**(8): 271–273.

21. Lins L, Carvalho FM. (2016) SF-36 total score as a single measure of health-related quality of life: Scoping review. *SAGE Open Med* **4**: 2050312116671725.

22. 国家中医药管理局. (1994) 中医病证诊断疗效标准.

23. 郑筱萸主编. (2002) 中药新药临床研究指导原则.

24. 国家中医药管理局. (2017) 国家中医药管理局办公室关于印发中风病 (脑梗死) 等 92 个病种中医临床路径和中医诊疗方案的通知 [EB/OL]. Available from: http://yzs.satcm.gov.cn/gongzuodongtai/2018-03-24/2651. html.

25. Tanaka Y, Kokubun S, Sato T. (1998) Mini-symposium: Cervical spine: (i) Cervical radiculopathy and its unsolved problems. *Curr Orthop* **12**(1): 1–6.

26. 姜宏, 施杞. (1996) 颈椎病疗效评定的研讨. *中国中医骨伤科杂志* **4**(4): 47–50.

27. 王晓红, 何成奇, 丁明甫, *et al.* (2005) 颈椎病治疗成绩评分表. 华西医学 **02**: 232–233.

28. 朱立国, 张清, 于杰, *et al.* (2009) 神经根型颈椎病疗效评定指标体系的效度分析. *中国中医骨伤科杂志* **17**(02): 22–23.

29. 张鸣生, 许伟成, 林仲民, 陈茵. (2003) 颈椎病临床评价量表的信度与效度研究. *中华物理医学与康复杂志* **25**(03): 25–28.

30. Schunemann H, Brozek J, Guyatt G, Oxman A. (eds.) (2013) *GRADE Handbook for Grading Quality of Evidence and Strength of Recommendations* (GRADE Working Group). Retrieved from: www.guidelinedevelopment.org/handbook.

5

Clinical Evidence for Chinese Herbal Medicine

OVERVIEW

This chapter summarises the available clinical evidence of Chinese herbal medicine for cervical radiculopathy. Randomised controlled trials, non-randomised controlled clinical trials and non-controlled studies were identified by searching nine major English and Chinese electronic medical databases. Where appropriate, Chinese herbal medicine treatments have been pooled in meta-analyses to assess their overall effects for different outcome measures. The quality of evidence has also been evaluated to assess the strength of available data. Frequently used Chinese herbal medicine formulae and herbs are summarised.

Introduction

Chinese herbal medicines (CHM) for the treatment of cervical radiculopathy (CR) have been examined by clinical studies and published in scientific journals, both in China and internationally. As presented in Chapter 4, the Methods for Evaluating Clinical Evidence section, a rigorous literature search, data screening, extraction and analysis process was undertaken. This chapter presents the key findings in the following categories: An overview of the previous systematic reviews, randomised controlled trials (RCTs), non-randomised controlled clinical trials (CCTs), and non-controlled studies.

Previous Systematic Reviews

Four systematic reviews evaluating the efficacy and safety of oral CHM for CR were identified. Two were published in English,[1,2] and the other two were in Chinese.[3,4]

The Zhang *et al.* study[3] systematically reviewed the efficacy and safety of a commercialised oral CHM product, namely the *Jing fu kang* granule 颈复康颗粒. The main herbs contained in this formula are *huang qi* 黄芪, *dang shen* 党参, *dan shen* 丹参, *chuan xiong* 川芎, *hong hua* 红花, *bai shao* 白芍, *sheng di huang* 生地黄, *ru xiang* 乳香, *mo yao* 没药, *ge gen* 葛根, etc. Three RCTs were included in this review, two of them comparing CHM with pharmacotherapy and the other RCT comparing the *Jing fu kang* granule 颈复康颗粒 with oral CHM. The effective rate was the only outcome measure evaluated in this systematic review. Due to the variety of control therapies, pooling the three studies in a meta-analysis is not appropriate. In addition, all included RCTs suffer from methodological weaknesses. Therefore, the review authors did not draw any conclusion.

The Zhu *et al.* study[1] also systematically assessed a commercialised oral CHM product, namely the *Jing tong* granule 颈痛颗粒. The main herbs contained in this product are *san qi* 三七, *chuan xiong* 川芎, *yan hu suo* 延胡索, *qiang huo* 羌活, *bai shao* 白芍, *wei ling xian* 威灵仙 and *ge gen* 葛根. Two RCTs evaluating the add-on effects of the *Jing tong* granule to conventional therapies and one RCT comparing it with a placebo were included in this review. This review suggested that 28 days of oral CHM treatment was more effective than a placebo for reducing pain; however, this was shown by a single study without meta-analysis. Two RCTs showed positive add-on effects of adding oral CHM to conventional therapy, with meta-analysis evidence of the Visual Analogue Scale (VAS) and a single study's results on the Neck Disability Index (NDI). Using the Grading of Recommendations, Assessment, Development and Evaluations (GRADE) approach, the authors concluded the evidence level was "low".

Chen *et al.*'s study in 2018[4] systematically reviewed 10 RCTs that either compared the oral CHM formula *Huang qi gui zhi wu wu tang* 黄芪桂枝五物汤 with routine pharmacotherapy (*n* = 6) or evaluated the formula as an add-on therapy to *tuina* 推拿 therapy (*n* = 4). Of the RCTs comparing oral CHM with routine pharmacotherapy, the meta-analysis result showed that oral CHM achieved better effects in terms of total effective rate and pain VAS. On the other hand, this formula also achieved significant add-on effects to *tuina* 推拿 therapy. The authors concluded that there was promising evidence supporting the use of the oral CHM formula *Huang qi gui zhi wu wu tang* 黄芪桂枝五物汤, but there was a need for high-quality, large-sized RCTs to confirm these effects.

Lee *et al.*'s study in 2018 evaluated RCTs on the oral CHM formula *Gegen* decotion 葛根汤.[2] Five RCTs were included in this review, including the oral CHM *Gegen* decotion compared to conventional treatment (*n* = 1), a combination of oral CHM and conventional therapy compared with conventional treatment alone (*n* = 1), and a combination of oral CHM and acupuncture compared with acupuncture alone (*n* = 3). Meta-analysis showed that the combination of oral CHM and acupuncture achieved better effects on the responder rate compared with acupuncture alone. The authors concluded that the evidence supporting the effects of the *Gegen* decotion for CR was insufficient due to the small number of studies and low methodological quality.

Identification of Clinical Studies

A search of nine English and Chinese language databases identified 20,537 citations, of which 4,369 required full-text retrieval to determine a citation's eligibility for inclusion (Fig. 5.1). After the assessment based on rigorous inclusion criteria, 48 clinical studies, which evaluated CHM for CR, were included. Of these, 29 studies were RCTs (H1 to H29) and 19 were non-controlled studies (H30 to H48). CHM was administered orally (22 RCTs and 18 non-controlled studies) or topically (7 RCTs and 1 non-controlled study). The evidence of oral CHM and topical CHM are presented separately. RCTs were evaluated to assess the efficacy and safety of CHM for CR, and details from non-controlled studies are described. In addition, two studies were identified utilising interventions not commonly practised outside

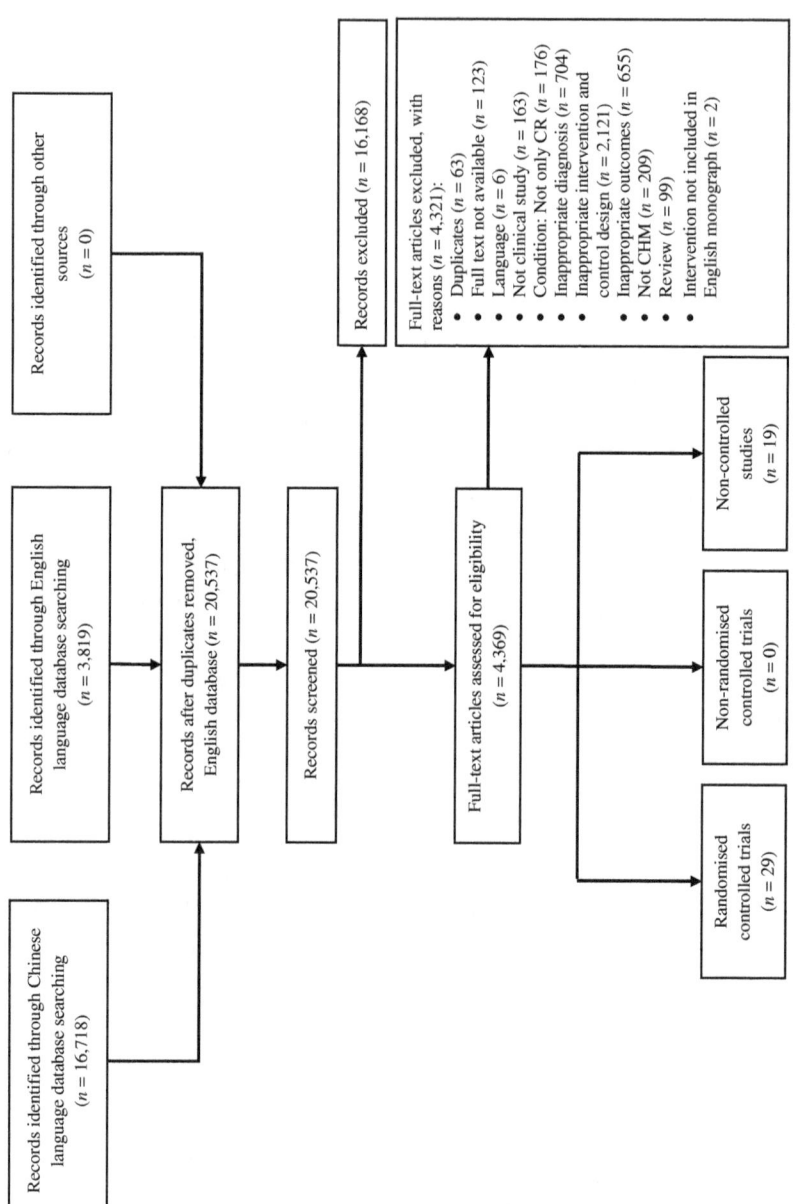

Fig. 5.1. Flow chart of study selection process: Chinese herbal medicine.

China; these studies are not presented here. The evidence on oral CHM and topical CHM is presented separately.

Randomised Controlled Trials of Oral Chinese Herbal Medicine

In total, 22 RCTs (H1 to H22) investigated oral CHM for CR in 1,833 participants. Participants included in these studies ranged from 25 to 70 years old (H5) and the duration of CR ranged from 15 days (H10) to 15 years (H5).

Of all the included studies, one RCT (H12) compared oral CHM with a placebo, nine RCTs (H1, H8, H13–18, H20) compared oral CHM with routine care that included pharmacotherapy and traction therapy, and 12 studies (H2–H7, H9–H11, H19, H21, H22) evaluated the add-on effects of oral CHM to some form of routine care.

The treatment duration ranged from two weeks (H1, H4, H5, H21) to 12 weeks (H20), with one month or four weeks being the most common treatment duration (H10–H12, H14, H18, H19).

Seven RCTs reported information on the Chinese medicine syndrome, with the most commonly seen syndromes being: *qi* stagnation and Blood stasis 气滞血瘀型 (H9, H19, H21) and wind-cold-dampness invasion 风寒湿型 (H5, H7, H18).

Of all included RCTs, six studies (H1, H11, H12, H15, H17, H20) evaluated commercialised CHM products that included pills, tablets or capsules. Six commercialised CHM products were evaluated by these studies, they are: *Bi qi jiao nang* 痹祺胶囊 (H1), *Jing tong ke li* 颈痛颗粒 (H11), *Qi she wan* 芪麝丸 (H12), *Shui zhi zhu yu jiao nang* 水蛭逐瘀胶囊, *Chuan ge shu jin wan* 川葛舒筋丸 (H15), *Teng huang jian gu pian* 藤黄健骨片 (H17), and *Gen tong ping ke li* (granules) 根痛平颗粒 (H20). The other 16 RCTs evaluated self-prescribed oral CHM formula decoctions, among which four studies (H6, H7, H10, H18) did not provide a formula name. Only one CHM formula, *Gui zhi jia ge gen tang* 桂枝加葛根汤, has been evaluated by multiple RCTs (H5–H7).

The routine care management used in these studies as comparators varied across studies, including traction therapy and nonsteroidal anti-inflammatory drugs (NSAIDs) (e.g., celecoxib, diclofenac, meloxicam and ibuprofen) and methylcobalamin.

Among all RCTs of oral CHM, the most frequently used herbs in products or decoctions were also analysed. See Table 5.1 for details.

Table 5.1. Frequently Reported Orally Used Herbs in Randomised Controlled Trials for Cervical Radiculopathy

Most Common Herb	Scientific Names	Frequency of Use
Ge gen 葛根	*Pueraria lobata* (Willd.) Ohwi	17
Bai shao 白芍/ Chi shao 赤芍	1. *Paeonia lactiflora* Pall. 2. *Paeonia veitchii* Lynch.	16 (13/3)
Gan cao 甘草	1. *Glycyrrhiza uralensis* Fisch. 2. *Glycyrrhiza inflata* Bat. 3. *Glycyrrhiza glabra* L.	14
Chuan xiong 川芎	*Ligusticum chuangxiong* Hort.	11
Gui zhi 桂枝	*Cinnamomum cassia* Presl.	10
Jiang 姜	*Zingiber officinale* Rosc.	8
Qiang huo 羌活	1. *Notopterygium incisum* Ting ex H.T. Chang 2. *Notopterygium franchetii* H. de Boiss.	8
Huang qi 黄芪	1. *Astragalus membranaceus* (Fisch.) Bge. var. mongholicus (Bge.) Hsiao 2. *Astragalus membranaceus* (Fisch.) Bge.	8
Di long 地龙	1. *Pheretima aspergillum* (E. Perrier) 2. *Pheretima vulgaris* Chen 3. *Pheretima guillelmi* (Michaelsen) 4. *Pheretima pectinifera* (Michaelsen)	7
Dang gui 当归	*Angelica sinensis* (Oliv.) Diels	7
Niu xi 牛膝	*Cyathula officinalis* Kuan	6
Dan shen 丹参	*Salvia miltiorrhiza* Bge.	5
Yan hu suo 延胡索	*Corydalis yanhusuo* W.T. Wang	5
Ji xue teng 鸡血藤	*Spatholobus suberectus* Dunn	5
Qin jiao 秦艽	1. *Gentiana macrophylla* Pall. 2. *Gentiana straminea* Maxim. 3. *Gentiana crassicaulis* Duthie ex Burk. 4. *Gentiana dahurica* Fisch.	4
Hong hua 红花	*Carthamus tinctorius* L.	4
Da zao 大枣	*Ziziphus jujuba* Mill.	3

Table 5.1. (*Continued*)

Most Common Herb	Scientific Names	Frequency of Use
Wei ling xian 威灵仙	1. *Clematis chinensis* Osbeck	3
	2. *Clematis hexapetala* Pall.	
	3. *Clematis manshurica* Rupr.	
Mo yao 没药	1. *Commiphora myrrha* Engl.	3
	2. *Commiphora molmol* Engl.	

Risk-of-Bias Assessment of Included Randomised Controlled Trials

Twelve RCTs did not report enough information to assess the risk of bias for sequence generation, and ten studies were rated at a "low" risk of bias as they reported using random number tables or computer-generated randomised numbers.

One study (H4) was assessed as a "high" risk for allocation concealment because the participant allocation was open to everyone in the study; two studies (H5, H12) were assessed as "low" risk for this domain since they used opaque envelopes to conceal the participant allocation; the other studies were all of "unclear" risk due to lack of information.

"Low" risk of bias for the blinding of participants, personnel and outcome assessor was achieved in one study (H12) with the use of a placebo CHM and effort in double-blinding. Others were at a "high" risk of bias for these three items since they applied different treatments in the intervention and control groups and did not apply any method to ensure blinding.

Two studies reported dropout cases without applying intention-to-treat method in their data analysis, but the low dropout rate was considered not to cause bias. The other studies did not have any dropouts. Hence, all studies were assessed as "low" risk of bias for the item of incomplete outcome data.

For selective reporting, two studies (H2, H10) were assessed as "high" risk of bias since they did not report the results of some

Table 5.2. Risk-of-Bias Assessment of Randomised Controlled Trials: Oral Chinese Herbal Medicine for Chronic Heart Failure Caused by Ischaemic Heart Disease

Risk-of-Bias Domain	Low Risk n (%)*	Unclear Risk n (%)*	High Risk n (%)*
Sequence generation	10 (45.5)	12 (54.5)	0 (0)
Allocation concealment	2 (9.1)	19 (86.4)	1 (4.5)
Blinding of participants	1 (4.5)	0 (0)	21 (95.5)
Blinding of personnel	1 (4.5)	0 (0)	21 (95.5)
Blinding of outcome assessors	1 (4.5)	0 (0)	21 (95.5)
Incomplete outcome data	22 (100)	0 (0)	0 (0)
Selective outcome reporting	0 (0)	20 (90.9)	2 (9.1)

*Percentage of total randomised controlled trials ($n = 22$).

outcomes defined in the methodology. Others were of "unclear" risk because they did not have the trial protocols registered or published. See Table 5.2 for a summary of the results.

Outcomes

Of all pre-defined outcome measures (see Chapter 4), the effective rate was the most commonly reported. It was reported in 15 studies (H1, H3–H6, H9, H11, H13–H18, H21, H22). The pain VAS or Numeric Rating Scale (NRS) was reported by 11 studies (H1, H4, H5, H8–H10, H12, H14, H17, H20, H21). In terms of specific CR outcome measures, three studies (H4, H9, H12) reported data on the NDI, seven studies (H1, H4, H5, H7, H11, H14, H19) reported data on the Scoring System for Cervical Radiculopathy (SSCR), one study (H18) used the Clinical Assessment Scale for Cervical Spondylosis (CASCS) and one study (H19) used the Outcome Assessment System in the Treatment of Cervical Radiculopathy (OASTCR). In addition, one study (H12) assessed patients' quality of life using the Short Form (36) Health Survey (SF-36).

The efficacy results are next presented under each comparison type and outcome.

Oral Chinese Herbal Medicine *vs.* Placebo

One thesis (H12) partially reported results of a multi-centre, double-blinded RCT comparing the oral CHM *Qi she* pill 芪麝丸 to a placebo. A total of 240 participants were included in this multi-centre RCT at a 1:1 ratio (120 *vs.* 120). The placebo was manufactured with the same appearance as the real CHM. All participants took either CHM or a placebo once a day for 28 days. Participants also had three- and six-month follow-up assessments after the treatment phase. The outcome measures used in this study were the pain VAS, NDI, SF-36 and adverse events (AEs). Huang's article in 2014 reported results for 48 participants (24 *vs.* 24) from one research centre. All participants completed the treatment, while three participants dropped out during the follow-up phase. Results showed that oral CHM was superior to the placebo at the end of the treatment phase for changes in the NDI, pain VAS and five domains of the SF-36 questionnaire (physical functioning bodily pain, social role functioning, emotional role functioning and vitality domains). Using an intention-to-treat (ITT) approach to address the dropouts, results showed that oral CHM was more effective than a placebo for NDI and pain VAS. Three mild cases of adverse events (AEs) occurred in the treatment group without medical treatment being required.

Oral Chinese Herbal Medicine *vs.* Routine Care Therapies

Nine studies compared oral CHM with routine care therapies, including pharmacotherapy (H1, H8, H14, H16, H17, H20), traction therapy (H15, H18) and a combination of pharmacotherapy and traction therapy (H13). Treatment effects are shown in Table 5.3, where meta-analysis was available.

Effective Rate

Using the effective rate to evaluate the treatment effects, meta-analysis results from eight RCTs showed that oral CHM was more

Table 5.3.   Oral Chinese Herbal Medicine *vs.* Routine Care Therapies

Outcome	Comparison	No. of Studies (Participants)	Effect Size (RR or MD: [95% CI], I²)	Included Studies
Effective rate	**Overall: Oral CHM *vs.* routine care therapies**	**8 (749)**	**RR: 1.14 [1.04, 1.24]*, 46%**	H1, H13–H15, H16–H18, H20
	Subgroup: Oral CHM *vs.* pharmacotherapy	5 (469)	RR: 1.11 [0.97, 1.26]*, 59%	H1, H14, H16, H17, H20
	Subgroup: Oral CHM *vs.* traction therapy	2 (210)	RR: 1.18 [1.06, 1.32]*, 0%	H15, H18
VAS/NRS	Oral CHM *vs.* pharmacotherapy	5 (493)	MD: −0.16 [−0.71, 0.40], 88%	H1, H8, H14, H17, H20
SSCR	Oral CHM *vs.* pharmacotherapy	2 (196)	MD: 2.87 [0.34, 5.41]*, 92%	H1, H14

Abbreviations: CHM, Chinese herbal medicine; CI, confidence interval; MD, mean difference; NRS, Numeric Rating Scale; RR, risk ratio; SSCR, Scoring System for Cervical Radiculopathy; VAS, Visual Analogue Scale.
*Statistically significant.

effective than routine care therapies (8 studies, RR: 1.14 [1.04, 1.24], I² = 46%). Subgrouping the studies according to the routine care therapies, it was found that oral CHM was more effective than pharmacotherapy (5 studies, RR: 1.11 [0.97, 1.26], I² = 59%) and traction therapy (2 studies, RR: 1.18 [1.06, 1.32], I² = 0%).

In addition, one study, including 70 participants, compared oral CHM with a combination of pharmacotherapy and traction therapy, and the effects based on the effective rate favoured CHM (RR, 1.28 [1.01, 1.62]) (H13).

Visual Analogue Scale/Numeric Rating Scale

In terms of pain assessed by the VAS or NRS, it was found that there was no significant difference between oral CHM and pharmacotherapy (5 studies, MD: −0.16 [−0.71, 0.40], I² = 88%).

Scoring System for Cervical Radiculopathy

Two studies comparing oral CHM with pharmacotherapy reported data on the SSCR and their results favoured oral CHM treatment (2 studies, MD: 2.87 [0.34, 5.41], I² = 92%).

Clinical Assessment Scale for Cervical Spondylosis

One study (H18) used the CASCS to evaluate the treatment effects of oral CHM compared with traction therapy, and the result favoured oral CHM (MD: 8.64 [5.22, 12.06]).

Oral Chinese Herbal Medicine Plus Routine Care Therapies *vs.* Routine Care Therapies

Twelve studies evaluated the add-on effects of oral CHM by comparing a combination of oral CHM and routine care therapies with routine care therapies alone. Eight (H2, H3, H6, H7, H9, H11, H19, H22) of these used traction therapy as the comparator, three studies (H4, H5, H10) used a combination of pharmacotherapy and traction therapy, and one study (H21) used pharmacotherapy as the comparator. The meta-analysis results of these studies are shown in Table 5.4.

Table 5.4. Oral Chinese Herbal Medicine Plus Routine Care Therapies *vs.* Routine Care Therapies

Outcome	Comparison	No. of Studies (Participants)	Effect Size (RR or MD: [95% CI], I^2)	Included Studies
Effective rate	Overall: Oral CHM add-on to routine care therapies	11 (913)	RR: 1.17 [1.11, 1.24]*, 0%	H2–7, H9, H11, H19, H21, H22
	Subgroup: Oral CHM add-on to traction therapy	8 (723)	RR: 1.20 [1.13, 1.28]*, 0%	H2, H3, H6, H7, H9, H11, H19, H22
	Subgroup: Oral CHM add-on to pharmacotherapy and traction therapy	2 (106)	RR: 1.00 [0.84, 1.19], 0%	H4, H5
VAS/NRS	Overall: Oral CHM add-on to routine care therapies	5 (303)	MD: −0.94 [−1.71, −0.18]*, 91%	H4, H5, H9, H10
	Subgroup: Oral CHM add-on to pharmacotherapy and traction therapy	3 (156)	MD: −0.49 [−0.93, −0.05]*, 30%	H4, H5, H10

(Continued)

Table 5.4. (*Continued*)

Outcome	Comparison	No. of Studies (Participants)	Effect Size (RR or MD: [95% CI], I²)	Included Studies
NDI	Overall: Oral CHM add-on to routine care therapies	2 (110)	MD: −2.89 [−8.73, 2.95]*, 97%	H4, H9
SSCR	Overall: Oral CHM add-on to routine care therapies	5 (291)	MD: 1.16 [0.21, 2.12]*, 68%	H4–H5, H7, H11, H19
	Subgroup: Oral CHM add-on to traction therapy	3 (185)	MD: 1.83 [0.44, 3.22]*, 66%	H7, H11, H19
	Subgroup: Oral CHM add-on to pharmacotherapy and traction therapy	2 (106)	MD: 0.23 [−0.48, 0.95], 0%	H4, H5

CHM: Chinese herbal medicine; CI: confidence interval; MD: mean difference; NDI: neck disability index; NRS: numeric rating scale; RR: risk ratio; SSCR: Scoring System for Cervical Radiculopathy; VAS: Visual Analogue Scale.
*Statistically significant.

Effective Rate

Assessed with the effective rate as the outcome measure, adding oral CHM to routine care was significantly more effective than routine care alone (11 studies, RR: 1.17 [1.11, 1.24], I² = 0%). By subgrouping these studies according to the comparator, it was found that adding oral CHM to traction therapy was superior to traction therapy alone (8 studies, RR: 1.20 [1.13, 1.28], I² = 0%). This superior effect was not found in the other subgroups.

It is worth mentioning that one study (H2) reported this outcome in a follow-up phase. This study reported that during the one-month post-treatment follow-up phase, the treatment effects for the oral CHM group were maintained in terms of the effective rate while the control group (traction therapy only) had one case of recurrence. This study concluded that adding oral CHM to traction therapy was beneficial for prolonged treatment effects.

Visual Analogue Scale/Numeric Rating Scale

Five studies reported data on pain using the VAS/NRS as the outcome measure. The overall meta-analysis showed that a combination of oral CHM and routine care therapies was superior to routine care therapies alone for pain scores (5 studies, MD: −0.94 [−1.71, −0.18], I^2 = 91%). Subgroup analysis confirmed that adding oral CHM to a combination of pharmacotherapy and traction therapy was beneficial (3 studies, MD: −0.49 [−0.93, −0.05], I^2 = 30%).

In addition, two RCTs evaluated the add-on effects of oral CHM to traction therapy (H9) and pharmacotherapy (H21), respectively, and the results of both studies showed a benefit of adding oral CHM for pain.

Neck Disability Index

The NDI was reported by two studies (H4, H9), with meta-analysis results showing significant add-on effects of oral CHM (2 studies, MD: −2.89 [−8.73, 2.95], I^2 = 97%).

Scoring System for Cervical Radiculopathy

Five studies (H4, H5, H7, H11, H19) reported data on the SSCR and their meta-analyses showed that adding oral CHM to routine care therapies was significantly more effective than routine care therapies alone (5 studies, MD: 1.16 [0.21, 2.12], I^2 = 68%). Subgroup analyses showed that adding oral CHM was beneficial for traction therapy (3 studies, MD: 1.83 [0.44, 3.22], I^2 = 66%), but not for a combination of pharmacotherapy and traction therapy (2 studies, MD: 0.23 [−0.48, 0.95], I^2 = 0%).

Outcome Assessment System in the Treatment of Cervical Radiculopathy

Only one study reported data on the OASTCR. Results showed that adding oral CHM to traction therapy was more effective than traction therapy alone (H19).

In addition, two studies (H4, H5) reported data on follow-up phases. Wei's study (H4) in 2017 reported data on the VAS, NDI and SSCR at the end of a two-week follow-up phase and there was no significant difference between the two groups for all three outcomes at the end of the follow-up. Ding's study (H5) in 2016 assessed the recurrence rate at the end of a three-month follow-up phase and reported that the CHM group had fewer recurrent cases than the pharmacotherapy group.

Assessment Using Grading of Recommendations Assessment, Development and Evaluation

The certainty of the evidence for oral CHM is presented in Tables 5.5 to 5.8, with two GRADE tables presenting the certainty of the evidence for oral CHM in comparison with routine care therapies (Tables 5.5 and 5.6) and the other two tables (Tables 5.7 and 5.8) presenting the certainty of the add-on effects of oral CHM, as below:

- Comparing oral CHM with pharmacotherapy, the evidence of the effective rate was of "moderate" certainty, while the evidence of the pain VAS and SSCR was of "low" or "very low" certainty;
- Comparing oral CHM with traction therapy, the certainty of evidence for the effective rate and CASCS was "low";
- Using oral CHM as an add-on therapy to traction therapy, the evidence of the effective rate was of "moderate" certainty, while the evidence of all other outcome measures was of "low" certainty; and
- Using oral CHM as an add-on therapy to traction therapy plus pharmacotherapy, the evidence of all outcome measures was of "low" certainty.

Among this evidence, the numbers of included studies and participants for most outcome measures were small (except for the effective rate) and the lack of blinding in the design of RCTs downgraded the certainty of their evidence.

Table 5.5.   GRADE: Oral Chinese Herbal Medicine *vs.* Pharmacotherapy

Outcome (End of Treatment)	Absolute Effect		Relative Effect (95% CI) No. of Participants (Studies)	Certainty of Evidence (GRADE)
	Oral CHM	**Pharmacotherapy**		
Effective rate	**89** per 100	**80** per 100	**RR 1.11** (0.97, 1.26)	⊕⊕⊕◯ MODERATE[1]
	Difference: 9 more per 100 patients (95% CI: 2 fewer to 21 more per 100 patients)		469 (5 RCTs)	
VAS/NRS	**2.74**	**2.90**	**MD −0.16** (−0.71, 0.4)	⊕⊕◯◯ LOW[1,3]
	Average difference: 0.16 lower (95% CI: 0.71 lower to 0.4 higher)		493 (5 RCTs)	
SSCR	**12.16**	**9.29**	**MD 2.87** (0.34, 5.41)	⊕◯◯◯ VERY LOW[1,2,3]
	Average difference: 2.87 higher (95% CI: 0.34 higher to 5.41 higher)		196 (2 RCTs)	

The risk in the intervention group (and its 95% CI) is based on the assumed risk in the comparison group and the relative effect of the intervention (and its 95% CI).

Abbreviations: CHM, Chinese herbal medicine; CI, confidence interval; GRADE, Grading of Recommendations Assessment, Development and Evaluation; MD, mean difference; NRS, numeric rating scale; SSCR, Scoring System for Cervical Radiculopathy; RCT, randomised controlled trial; RR, risk ratio; VAS, Visual Analogue Scale.

Notes:
1) Lack of blinding of participants and personnel may have influenced results;
2) Small sample sizes may have limited the certainty of results; and
3) High heterogeneity may have limited the certainty of results.

Study references:
Effective rate: H1, H14, H16, H17, H20
VAS/NRS: H1, H8, H14, H17, H20
SSCR: H1, H14

Frequently Reported Orally Used Herbs in Meta-Analyses Showing Favourable Effect for Cervical Radiculopathy

The most frequent herbs used in studies from favourable meta-analyses were calculated (Table 5.9). Studies were pooled according to the

Table 5.6. GRADE: Oral Chinese Herbal Medicine *vs.* Traction Therapy

Outcome (End of Treatment)	Absolute Effect		Relative Effect (95% CI) No. of Participants (Studies)	Certainty of Evidence (GRADE)
	Oral CHM	Traction Therapy		
Effective rate	93 per 100	79 per 100	RR 1.18 (1.06, 1.32)	⊕⊕◯◯ LOW[1,2]
	Difference: 14 more per 100 patients (95% CI: 5 more to 25 more per 100 patients)		210 (2 RCTs)	
CASCS	95.41	86.77	MD 8.64 (5.22, 12.06)	⊕⊕◯◯ LOW[1,2]
	Average difference: 8.64 higher (95% CI: 5.22 higher to 12.06 higher)		110 (1 RCT)	

The risk in the intervention group (and its 95% CI) is based on the assumed risk in the comparison group and the relative effect of the intervention (and its 95% CI).

Abbreviations: CASCS, Clinical Assessment Scale for Cervical Spondylosis; CHM, Chinese herbal medicine; CI, confidence interval; GRADE, Grading of Recommendations Assessment, Development and Evaluation; MD, mean difference; RCT, randomised controlled trial; RR, risk ratio.

Notes:
1) Lack of blinding of participants and personnel may have influenced results;
2) Small sample sizes may have limited the certainty of results; and
3) High heterogeneity may have limited the certainty of results.

Study references:
Effective rate: H15, H18
CASCS: H18

main outcome measure groups regardless of their comparator (CHM *vs.* routine care or CHM add-on to routine care):

- There were two meta-analyses of the effective rate showing positive results; 19 RCTs were included in these two meta-analyses. A total of 63 herbs were used in these studies, the most common being *bai shao* 白芍/*chi shao* 赤芍/*shao yao* 芍药, *ge gen* 葛根, *gan cao* 甘草 and *gui zhi* 桂枝, which were used in more than half of the studies; and

Table 5.7. GRADE: Oral Chinese Herbal Medicine Plus Traction Therapy *vs.* Traction Therapy

Outcome (End of Treatment)	Absolute Effect		Relative Effect (95% CI) No. of Participants (Studies)	Certainty of Evidence (GRADE)
	Oral CHM Plus Traction Therapy	Traction Therapy		
Effective rate	90 per 100	75 per 100	RR 1.20 (1.13, 1.28)	⊕⊕⊕◯ MODERATE[1]
	Difference: 15 more per 100 patients (95% CI: 10 more to 21 more per 100 patients)		723 (8 RCTs)	
VAS/NRS	1.86	3.95	MD −2.09 (−2.46, −1.72)	⊕⊕◯◯ LOW[1,2]
	Average difference: 2.09 lower (95% CI: 2.46 lower to 1.72 lower)		63 (1 RCT)	
NDI	17.06	22.98	MD −5.92 (−7.68, −4.16)	⊕⊕◯◯ LOW[1,2]
	Average difference: 5.92 lower (95% CI: 7.68 lower to 4.16 lower)		63 (1 RCT)	
SSCR	14.22	12.39	MD 1.83 (0.44, 3.22)	⊕⊕◯◯ LOW[1,2]
	Average difference: 1.83 higher (95% CI: 0.44 higher to 3.22 higher)		185 (3 RCTs)	
OASTCR	5.23	6.14	MD −0.91 (−1.44, −0.38)	⊕⊕◯◯ LOW[1,2]
	Average difference: 0.91 lower (95% CI: 1.44 lower to 0.38 lower)		70 (1 RCT)	

The risk in the intervention group (and its 95% CI) is based on the assumed risk in the comparison group and the relative effect of the intervention (and its 95% CI).

Abbreviations: CHM, Chinese herbal medicine; CI, confidence interval; GRADE, Grading of Recommendations Assessment, Development and Evaluation; MD, mean difference; NDI, neck disability index; NRS, numeric rating scale; OASTCR, Outcome Assessment System in the Treatment of Cervical Radiculopathy; RCT, randomised controlled trial; RR, risk ratio; SSCR, Scoring System for Cervical Radiculopathy; VAS, Visual Analogue Scale.

Notes:
1) Lack of blinding of participants and personnel may have influenced results;
2) Small sample sizes may have limited the certainty of results; and
3) High heterogeneity may have limited the certainty of results.

Study references:
Effective rate: H2, H3, H6, H7, H9, H11, H19, H22
VAS/NRS: H9
NDI: H9
SSCR: H7, H11, H19
OASTCR: H19

119

Table 5.8. GRADE: Oral Chinese Herbal Medicine Plus Pharmacotherapy Plus Traction Therapy *vs.* Pharmacotherapy Plus Traction Therapy

Outcome (End of Treatment)	Absolute Effect		Relative Effect (95% CI) No. of Participants (Studies)	Certainty of Evidence (GRADE)
	Oral CHM plus Pharmacotherapy Plus Traction Therapy	Pharmacotherapy Plus Traction Therapy		
Effective rate	83 per 100	83 per 100	RR 1.00 (0.84, 1.19)	⊕⊕◯◯ LOW[1,2]
	Difference: 0 higher or lower per 100 patients (95% CI: 13 fewer to 16 more per 100 patients)		106 (2 RCT)	
VAS/NRS	1.69 per 100	2.18 per 100	MD −0.49 (−0.93, −0.05)	⊕⊕◯◯ LOW[1,2]
	Average difference: 0.49 lower (95% CI: 0.93 lower to 0.05 lower)		156 (3 RCTs)	
NDI	6.21	6.17	MD 0.04 (−0.80, 0.88)	⊕⊕◯◯ LOW[1,2]
	Average difference: 0.04 higher (95% CI: 0.80 lower to 0.88 higher)		47 (1 RCTs)	
SSCR	11.49	11.26	MD 0.23 (−0.48, 0.95)	⊕⊕◯◯ LOW[1,2]
	Average difference: 0.23 higher (95% CI: 0.48 lower to 0.95 higher)		106 (2 RCT)	

The risk in the intervention group (and its 95% CI) is based on the assumed risk in the comparison group and the relative effect of the intervention (and its 95% CI).

Abbreviations: CHM, Chinese herbal medicine; CI, confidence interval; GRADE, Grading of Recommendations Assessment, Development and Evaluation; MD, mean difference; NDI, Neck Disability Index; NRS, numeric rating scale; OASTCR, Outcome Assessment System in the Treatment of Cervical Radiculopathy; RCT, randomised controlled trial; RR, risk ratio; SSCR, Scoring System for Cervical Radiculopathy; VAS, Visual Analogue Scale.

Notes:
1) Lack of blinding of participants and personnel may have influenced results;
2) Small sample sizes may have limited the certainty of results; and
3) High heterogeneity may have limited the certainty of results.

Study references:
Effective rate: H4, H5
VAS/NRS: H4, H5, H10
NDI: H4
SSCR: H4, H5

Table 5.9. Frequently Reported Orally Used Herbs in Meta-Analyses Showing Favourable Effect for Cervical Radiculopathy

Outcome Measure	No. of Meta-Analyses	No. of Studies	Herbs	Scientific Names	Frequency of Use
Effective rate	2	19	Bai shao 白芍/Chi shao 赤芍/Shao yao 芍药	1. *Paeonia lactiflora* Pall. 2. *Paeonia veitchii* Lynch	17
			Ge gen 葛根	*Pueraria lobata* (Willd.) Ohwi	15
			Gan cao 甘草	1. *Glycyrrhiza uralensis* Fisch. 2. *Glycyrrhiza inflata* Bat. 3. *Glycyrrhiza glabra* L.	13
			Gui zhi 桂枝	*Cinnamomum cassia* Presl.	10
			Chuan xiong 川芎	*Ligusticum chuangxiong* Hort.	9
			Jiang 姜	*Zingiber officinale* Rosc.	8
			Qiang huo 羌活	1. *Notopterygium incisum* Ting ex H.T. Chang 2. *Notopterygium franchetii* H. de Boiss.	7
			Dang gui 当归	*Angelica sinensis* (Oliv.) Diels	6
			Niu xi 牛膝	*Cyathula officinalis* Kuan	6
			Fu zi 附子/Wu tou 乌头	*Aconitum carmichaelii* Debx.	6
NDI and SSCR	3	8	Ge gen 葛根	*Pueraria lobata* (Willd.) Ohwi	7
			Gan cao 甘草	1. *Glycyrrhiza uralensis* Fisch. 2. *Glycyrrhiza inflata* Bat. 3. *Glycyrrhiza glabra* L.	5
			Bai shao 白芍	*Paeonia lactiflora* Pall.	5
			Yan hu suo 延胡索	*Corydalis yanhusuo* W.T. Wang	4
			Wu tou 乌头	*Aconitum carmichaelii* Debx.	4
			Dan shen 丹参	*Salvia miltiorrhiza* Bge.	4
			Chuan xiong 川芎	*Ligusticum chuangxiong* Hort.	4
			Gui zhi 桂枝	*Cinnamomum cassia* Presl.	4

(Continued)

Table 5.9. (*Continued*)

Outcome Measure	No. of Meta-Analyses	No. of Studies	Herbs	Scientific Names	Frequency of Use
			Qin jiao 秦艽	1. *Gentiana macrophylla* Pall.	3
				2. *Gentiana straminea* Maxim.	
				3. *Gentiana crassicaulis* Duthie ex Burk.	
				4. *Gentiana dahurica* Fisch.	

Abbreviations: NDI, neck disability index; SSCR, Scoring System for Cervical Radiculopathy.
Note: The use of some herbs such as *fu zi* 附子 and *wu tou* 乌头 may be restricted in some countries. Readers are advised to comply with relevant regulations.

- Three meta-analyses of CR-specific outcome measures (the NDI and SSCR) showed positive results with eight studies included. The herbs *ge gen* 葛根, *bai shao* 白芍, *gan cao* 甘草, *yan hu suo* 延胡索 and *wu tou* 乌头 were used in more than half the included studies.

Randomised Controlled Trial Evidence for Individual Oral Chinese Herbal Medicine Formulae

Among the included RCTs, the oral CHM formulae varied greatly across all studies. Only one oral CHM formula was evaluated by multiple studies: *Gui zhi jia ge gen tang* 桂枝加葛根汤, which was evaluated in three RCTs (H5–H7). Meta-analyses of these studies showed that adding this oral CHM formula to routine care was more effective than routine care when using the effective rate as the outcome measure (3 studies, RR: 1.16 [1.03, 1.30], $I^2 = 0\%$), but this positive result was not found with the SSCR (2 studies, 1.42 [−0.17, 3.00], $I^2 = 43\%$) (H5, H7). There was no meta-analysis result as evidence of other CHM formulae due to the diversity of the formulae and designs of studies.

Safety of Oral Chinese Herbal Medicine in Randomised Controlled Trials

Nine studies (H1, H4, H5, H8, H11, H12, H17, H19, H20) mentioned safety information. Among these, three studies (H11, H17,

H19) reported that there were no AEs observed. Six studies (H1, H4, H5, H8, H12, H20) reported AEs; the AEs that occurred in the oral CHM group were mainly mild gastrointestinal symptoms such as stomacheache, nausea and diarrhea, and did not require medical treatment.

Non-Controlled Studies of Oral Chinese Herbal Medicine

Seventeen non-controlled case series studies (H30–H40, H42–H47) and one case report (H41) were identified from our comprehensive search in reporting the effectiveness of oral CHM for the management of CR. A total of 3,130 patients were involved in these studies. The CHM formula *Huang qi gui zhi wu wu tang* 黄芪桂枝五物汤 with certain modifications was applied in three studies (H35, H41, H46) in a decoction form. The most common orally used herbs were: *huang qi* 黄芪 (*n* = 16), *bai shao* 白芍 (*n* = 13), *ge gen* 葛根 (*n* = 13), *gui zhi* 桂枝 (*n* = 12), *chuan xiong* 川芎 (*n* = 11), *dang gui* 当归 (*n* = 11), *hong hua* 红花 (*n* = 8), *sheng jiang* 生姜 (*n* = 7), *tao ren* 桃仁 (*n* = 6) and *ji xue teng* 鸡血藤 (*n* = 6).

The outcomes reported by these studies were the effective rate (H30–H36, H39, H40, H42, H44, H46, H47), VAS (H33, H42) and the McGill Pain Questionnaire (MPQ) (H33). Only one study (H33) mentioned that there were mild gastrointestinal symptoms caused by the CHM, while the other studies did not provide information on CHM safety.

Randomised Controlled Trials of Topical Chinese Herbal Medicine

Seven RCTs (H23–H29) investigated topical CHM for CR in 884 participants. Four studies (H23, H25, H26, H29) compared topical CHM with routine care, including pharmacotherapy and traction therapy, and three studies (H24, H27, H28) investigated the add-on effects of topical CHM to traction therapy. Participants included in these studies ranged from 36 to 70 years old (H1) and the duration of CR ranged from three days (H1) to eight years (H1).

The topical CHM were used in different forms: CHM ointments (H23, H24), CHM heat packs (H25, H26, H29) and CHM decoctions applied using an iontophoresis apparatus which assists the process of transdermal drug delivery (H27, H28). It is worth noting that the CHM heat pack therapy is also informally named "CHM ironing therapy", as pointed out by two studies (H25, H26).

A Chinese medicine syndrome differentiation approach was applied in two studies (H25, H26), indicating that the participants were diagnosed with *qi* stagnation and Blood stasis 气滞血瘀证 or wind-cold-dampness invasion 风寒湿证. One study (H25) applied different CHM treatments according to syndrome differentiation types. The CHM formulae used in the seven studies all varied, without any formula being evaluated by multiple studies. Three studies provided names of their topical CHM formulae as: *Ma qian zi yao gao* 马钱子药膏 (H23), *Tong luo zhi tong fang* 通络止痛方 (H24), and *Huo xue san* 活血散 (H26). One study (H27) applied CHM iontophoresis therapy using *Dang gui zhu she ye* 当归注射液. A total of 47 herbs were found in these studies, with *dang gui* 当归 (*n* = 4), *hong hua* 红花 (*n* = 4), *wei ling xian* 威灵仙 (*n* = 3), *chuan wu tou* 川乌头 (*n* = 3), and *qiang huo* 羌活 (*n* = 3) being the most common (see Table 5.10).

Risk-of-Bias Assessment of Included Randomised Controlled Trials

None of the seven RCTs reported sufficient information to assess the risk of bias for sequence generation; therefore they were all assessed as "unclear" risk for this item. One study (H27) applied the opaque-envelope concealing method and was assessed as "low" risk for allocation concealment; the other studies were of "unclear" risk for this item due to a lack of information. The blinding of participants, personnel and outcome assessors was not achieved in any of the included studies because they all applied different therapies for the intervention and control groups and did not make any efforts to attain

Table 5.10.   Frequently Reported Topically Used Herbs in Randomised Controlled Trials for Cervical Radiculopathy

Most Common Herbs	Scientific Names	Frequency of Use
Dang gui 当归	*Angelica sinensis* (Oliv.) Diels	4
Hong hua 红花	*Carthamus tinctorius* L.	4
Wu tou 乌头	*Aconitum carmichaelii* Debx.	3
Wei ling xian 威灵仙	1. *Clematis chinensis* Osbeck 2. *Clematis hexapetala* Pall. 3. *Clematis manshurica* Rupr.	3
Qiang huo 羌活	1. *Notopterygium incisum* Ting ex H. T. Chang 2. *Notopterygium franchetii* H. de Boiss.	3

Note: The use of some herbs such as *wu tou* 乌头 may be restricted in some countries. Readers are advised to comply with relevant regulations.

blinding. No studies had dropouts, so they were assessed as "low" risk of bias in incomplete outcome data. For selective reporting, one study (H26) was assessed as "high" risk of bias since it did not report results for some outcomes defined in the methodology, while the others were of "unclear" risk because none of these had their trial protocols registered or published. See Table 5.11 for a summary of the results.

Outcomes

Six RCTs (H23–H27, H29) reported data on the effective rate and two studies (H24, H25) reported data on the pain VAS/NRS. Liu's study (H27) in 2008 also reported data on the MPQ and OASTCR to evaluate the treatment effects. The efficacy results are next presented under each outcome and comparison type.

Topical Chinese Herbal Medicine *vs.* Routine Care Therapies

Four RCTs (H23, H25, H26, H29) compared topical CHM with routine care therapies, with one study (H23) comparing topical CHM with pharmacotherapy, one study (H25) comparing topical CHM with traction therapy, and two studies (H26, H29) comparing topical CHM with physical therapy.

Table 5.11.   Risk of Bias of Randomised Controlled Trials: Oral Chinese Herbal Medicine for Chronic Heart Failure Caused by Ischaemic Heart Disease

Risk of Bias Domain	Low Risk n (%)*	Unclear Risk n (%)*	High Risk n (%)*
Sequence generation	0 (0)	7 (100)	0 (0)
Allocation concealment	1 (14.3)	6 (85.7)	0 (0)
Blinding of participants	0 (0)	0 (0)	7 (100)
Blinding of personnel	0 (0)	0 (0)	7 (100)
Blinding of outcome assessors	0 (0)	0 (0)	7 (100)
Incomplete outcome data	7 (100)	0 (0)	0 (0)
Selective outcome reporting	0 (0)	6 (85.7)	1 (14.3)

*Percentage of total randomised controlled trials ($n = 7$).

Table 5.12.   Topical Chinese Herbal Medicine *vs.* Routine Care Therapies

Outcome	Comparison	No. of Studies (Participants)	Effect Size (RR or MD: [95% CI], I^2)	Included Studies
Effective rate	Overall: Topical CHM *vs.* routine care therapies	4 (620)	RR: 1.11 [0.98, 1.25], 71%	H23, H25, H26, H29
	Subgroup: Topical CHM *vs.* physical therapy	2 (160)	RR: 1.22 [0.95, 1.56], 67%	H26, H29

Abbreviations: CHM, Chinese herbal medicine; CI, confidence interval; MD, mean difference; RR, risk ratio.

Effective Rate

Four studies (H23, H25, H26, H29) reported data on the effective rate (Table 5.12). The overall analysis showed that there was no significant difference between topical CHM and routine care therapies (4 studies, 1.11 [0.98, 1.25], $I^2 = 71\%$). Grouping the studies according to the routine care therapies, it was found by subgroup analyses that the effective rate of topical CHM was not different with pharmacotherapy (H23), traction therapy (H25) or physical therapy (H26, H29).

Visual Analogue Scale

Only one study (H25) used the pain VAS to evaluate the treatment effects, showing that the topical CHM heat pack therapy was more effective than traction therapy for pain relief.

In addition, one study (H26) assessed the effective rate, symptom scores and patients' cervical range of motion (ROM) at the end of a 45-day follow-up phase. It was reported that at the end of the follow-up phase, the CHM group achieved better effects than the physiotherapy group for all these outcomes.

Topical Chinese Herbal Medicine Plus Routine Care Therapies *vs.* Routine Care Therapies

Three studies (H24, H27, H28) evaluated the add-on effects of topical CHM to traction therapy. One study (H24) used CHM external application and the other two studies (H27, H28) used iontophoresis apparatus for topical CHM delivery.

Using the effective rate to assess the treatment effects, overall meta-analysis showed the superior effects of adding topical CHM to traction therapy (3 studies, RR: 1.23 [1.08, 1.40], $I^2 = 27\%$) (H24, H27, H28). One study (H24) reported data on the pain VAS and superior effects of adding topical CHM to traction therapy was found (MD: −1.23 [−1.80, −0.66]. One study (H27) reported data on the MPQ and a significant benefit was obtained (MD: −1.26 [−2.24, −0.28].

Assessment Using Grading of Recommendations Assessment, Development and Evaluation

The certainty of evidence for topical CHM being used as an add-on therapy is presented in Table 5.13. There was only a single study that provided evidence of the effective rate and pain VAS, in which

Table 5.13. GRADE: Topical Chinese Herbal Medicine Plus Traction Therapy *vs.* Traction Therapy

Outcome (End of Treatment)	Absolute Effect		Relative Effect (95% CI) No. of Participants (Studies)	Certainty of Evidence (GRADE)
	Topical CHM Plus Traction Therapy	**Traction Therapy**		
Effective rate	**93** per 100	**70** per 100	**RR 1.33** (1.04, 1.72)	⊕⊕○○ LOW[1,2]
	Average difference: 23 more per 100 patients (95% CI: 3 more to 50 more per 100 patients)		60 (1 RCT)	
VAS/NRS	**1.87**	**3.10**	**MD −1.23** (−1.80, −0.66)	⊕⊕○○ LOW[1,2]
	Average difference: 1.23 lower (95% CI: 1.80 lower to 0.66 lower)		60 (1 RCT)	

The risk in the intervention group (and its 95% CI) is based on the assumed risk in the comparison group and the relative effect of the intervention (and its 95% CI).

Abbreviations: CHM, Chinese herbal medicine; CI, confidence interval; GRADE, Grading of Recommendations Assessment, Development and Evaluation; MD, mean difference; NRS, numeric rating scale; RCT, randomised controlled trial; RR, risk ratio; VAS, Visual Analogue Scale.

Notes:
1) Lack of blinding of participants and personnel may have influenced results;
2) Small sample sizes may have limited the certainty of results; and
3) High heterogeneity may have limited the certainty of results.

Study references:
Effective rate: H24
VAS/NRS: H24

topical CHM was used as an add-on therapy to traction therapy; both of these two outcomes were assessed as "low" certainty evidence. The small sample size and lack of blinding downgraded the certainty of this evidence.

Frequently Reported Topically Used Herbs in Meta-Analyses Showing Favourable Effect for Cervical Radiculopathy

There were two meta-anlyses of the effective rate that showed positive results. Seven studies were included in these two meta-analyses,

Table 5.14. Frequently Reported Topically Used Herbs in Meta-Analyses Showing Favourable Effect for Cervical Radiculopathy

Outcome Measure	No. of Meta-Analyses	No. of Studies	Herbs	Scientific Names	Frequency of Use
Effective rate	2	7	Fu zi 附子/Wu tou 乌头	*Aconitum carmichaelii* Debx.	5
			Wei ling xian 威灵仙	1. *Clematis chinensis* Osbeck 2. *Clematis hexapetala* Pall. 3. *Clematis manshurica* Rupr.	4
			Dang gui 当归	*Angelica sinensis* (Oliv.) Diels	4
			Hong hua 红花	*Carthamus tinctorius* L.	4
			Qiang huo 羌活	1. *Notopterygium incisum* Ting ex H.T. Chang 2. *Notopterygium franchetii* H. de Boiss.	3

Note: The use of some herbs such as *fu zi* 附子 and *wu tou* 乌头 may be restricted in some countries. Readers are advised to comply with relevant regulations.

with a total of 44 different herbs being used. The herbs *fu zi* 附子/*wu tou* 乌头, *wei ling xian* 威灵仙, *dang gui* 当归, and *hong hua* 红花 were used in more than half of the included studies (Table 5.14).

Randomised Controlled Trial Evidence for Individual Topical Chinese Herbal Medicine Formulae

Due to the small number of included studies and the diversity of topical CHM formulae and their administrative methods, there was no topical CHM formula evaluated by multiple RCTs. Therefore, meta-analysis evidence to confirm the efficacy of individual topical CHM formulae is lacking in our evaluation.

Safety of Topical Chinese Herbal Medicine in Randomised Controlled Trials

Safety information was reported by five studies (H23–H26, H29). Three studies (H24, H25, H29) suggested that there were no adverse events (AEs) observed in the studies. Two studies reported mild skin irritation and allergy caused by the topical CHM (H23, H26) without additional medical care needed.

Non-Controlled Studies of Topical Chinese Herbal Medicine

One non-controlled case series study (H48) reported the effects of an externally used CHM heat pack on 50 patients. In this study, 14 herbs were ground into powder, then mixed with coarse salt and packaged into a heat pack. The heat pack was applied on the neck region twice a day for 15 days. The effective rate and VAS were chosen to assess the treatment's effects.

Evidence for Chinese Herbal Medicine Treatments Commonly Used in Clinical Practice

The common practices of CHM treatments for CR recommended by guidelines and textbooks are summarised in Chapter 2. Many of the formulae recommended for CR in Chapter 2 have not been evaluated in clinical studies. Pooling all types of clinical studies, it was found that five oral CHM formulae have been evaluated by multiple studies:

- *Gui zhi jia ge gen tang* 桂枝加葛根汤 has been evaluated by three RCTs (H5–H7);
- *Ge gen tang* 葛根汤 was evaluated by one RCT (H3) and one non-controlled study (H32);
- *Jing tong ke li* 颈痛颗粒 was also evaluated by one RCT (H11) and one non-controlled study (H39);
- *Huang qi gui zhi wu wu tang* 黄芪桂枝五物汤 has evidence from three non-controlled studies (H35, H41, H46); and
- *Jin bi fang* 筋痹方 was reported by two non-controlled studies (H36, H47).

Among all the CHM formulae recommended in Chapter 2, only two oral CHM formulae have clinical research evidence: *Shen tong zhu yu tang* 身痛逐瘀汤, which was evaluated by one RCT (H13) but it was used in combination with another CHM formula in this study; and *Huang qi gui zhi wu wu tang* 黄芪桂枝五物汤, which was reported in three non-controlled studies (H35, H41, H46). Therefore, there is no meta-analysis result supporting the efficacy of the oral CHM formulae recommended in Chapter 2.

In terms of topically used CHM formulae, only one CHM product used via iontophoresis has been assessed by an RCT: *Dang gui zhu she ye* 当归注射液 (H27).

Although the other formulae may have not been titled with commonly known CHM formula names, their treatment principles based on syndrome differentiation and ingredients are similar to those suggested in Chapter 2.

Summary of Chinese Herbal Medicine Clinical Evidence

The evaluation of clinical studies found variation in terms of the formulae of CHM and diversity in the outcomes reported. There was more clinical evidence supporting the use of oral CHM than topical CHM.

The ages of participants in all included clinical studies ranged from 20 to 70 years old with most participants around 50 years of age, which is consistent with the common age of onset of this disease. The duration of disease ranged from days to eight years, but it was not possible to conduct subgroup analysis based on disease duration due to the limitations in data reporting. A Chinese medicine syndrome differentiation approach was incorporated in both oral CHM and topical CHM treatments, but only in a relatively small number of studies. Among these, the syndromes of *qi* stagnation and Blood stasis 气滞血瘀证 and wind-cold-dampness invasion 风寒湿证 were the most common ones reported.

A number of different forms of CHM were used in the clinical studies included in the evaluation of this monograph. Oral CHM was delivered as decoctions, granules, tablets or capsules. Topical CHM was administered as ointments or heat packs, or via CHM bathing or steaming, CHM iontophoresis, etc. The CHM formulae evaluated by the included clinical studies varied, with only one oral CHM formula (*Gui zhi jia ge gen tang* 桂枝加葛根汤 being assessed by multiple RCTs and the meta-analysis result supporting its add-on effects in terms of overall benefit. A topical CHM formula used as a heat pack for topical application, coarse salt 粗盐 in combination with other herbs, was assessed by one RCT and one non-controlled study. In China, some CHM formulae or single-herb extractions are made as intravenous (IV) solutions. The IV CHMs are commonly administered in clinical practice in China but are not covered in this monograph. It is worth noting that the IV CHM solutions can also be administered as topical CHM through skin absorption, although meta-analysis of this practice is lacking.

In the included clinical studies, the treatment duration ranged from seven days to 90 days. A four-week or one-month-long treatment duration was very common in oral CHM treatment, while topical CHM usually was applied for two weeks. It seems that topical CHM was administered for a shorter duration than oral CHM. This may be explained by the procedure of administration, as applying topical CHM involves certain equipment (e.g., iontophoresis apparatus) or complicated procedures, while the administration of oral CHM is simpler, such as oral CHM granules, tablets or capsules. Our evaluation of RCTs revealed that the add-on effects of topical CHM to routine care was significant, but with a very small number of studies included in the meta-analysis.

The effects of CHM treatment were evidenced by meta-analyses, including:

- Oral CHM was more effective than routine care in terms of the effective rate (meta-analyses of two RCTs) and SSCR (meta-analyses of two RCTs);
- Oral CHM plus routine care was more effective than routine care alone in terms of the effective rate (meta-analyses of 11 RCTs), the pain VAS/NRS (meta-analyses of five RCTs), the NDI (meta-analyses of two RCTs) and the SSCR (meta-analyses of five RCTs); and
- Topical CHM was more effective than routine care in terms of the effective rate (meta-analyses of three RCTs).

As assessed by the GRADE approach, the certainty of most of the evidence was "low". Only the evidence of the effective rate was of "moderate certainty". It is worth pointing out that the small sample sizes and lack of blinding downgraded the certainty of most evidence.

On the other hand, whether any effects of CHM could extend after the treatment phase was unclear, since most of the studies did not include a follow-up phase to evaluate the long-term effects.

Considering that the CHM formulae used in the clinical studies varied greatly, it was difficult to discover effective formulae based on our evaluation. The method of pooling all studies was included in positive meta-analyses. We then summarised the frequently used herbs from these studies. It was found that *shao yao* 芍药 (including *bai shao* 白芍, *chi shao* 赤芍 or *shao yao* 芍药, *ge gen* 葛根, *gan cao* 甘草, *chuan xiong* 川芎, *fu zi* 附子/*wu tou* 乌头 and *gui zhi* 桂枝 were the orally used herbs that appeared in the positive meta-analyses in included studies with pools of two types of outcome measure, while the herbs *fu zi* 附子/*wu tou* 乌头, *wei ling xian* 威灵仙, *dang gui* 当归, and *hong hua* 红花 may have been effective for topical application. It should be pointed out that *fu zi* (附子 and *wu tou* 乌头 are commonly used for pain relief but they may be restricted in some countries, so readers are advised to consider the toxicity of these herbs and comply with relevant regulations.

In terms of the safety of CHM therapy, there were no severe AEs reported by the included clinical studies. Only mild gastrointestinal symptoms caused by oral CHM and mild skin irritation and allergy caused by topical CHM were mentioned in a small number of studies. Furthermore, due to the lack of long-term follow-up in most studies, it is not possible to conclude whether there were any delayed noticeable AEs of CHM.

Among the controlled studies, only one study compared CHM with a placebo. The other studies were designed to either compare CHM with routine care therapies or compare a combination of CHM and routine care therapies with routine care therapies alone. All the included clinical studies were conducted in China and recruited participants from hospitals. Chinese medicine has a long history of practice in China and it is a part of the traditional culture among the Chinese population, so it is not surprising that the people who seek CHM treatment hold a strong belief in Chinese medicine therapies. Therefore, without an appropriate placebo control, the potential placebo effects of these therapies could not be ruled out. Readers should interpret the above-mentioned treatment effect results with caution.

It is also important to note that the quality of reporting of the included studies was low. Most studies did not provide subgroup results based on the disease baseline severity or duration, Chinese medicine syndrome type or age. Therefore, it was not possible to conduct subgroup meta-analyses taking these factors into consideration.

In addition, the outcome measures used in these studies were not entirely consistent with what are recommended by international clinical guidelines. As introduced in Chapter 4, the NDI, SF-36 (or SF-12), pain VAS and NRS are recommended by international clinical guidelines; among these, the pain VAS or NRS were commonly reported, but the NDI and SF-36 (or SF-12) were seldom reported. On the other hand, there were some outcome measures commonly seen in studies conducted in China, such as the effective rate, SSCR and OASTCR. Of these, the effective rate (reported by 40 out of 48 studies) and pain VAS/NRS (reported by 17 out of 48 studies) were the most commonly reported. The NDI was used in only three RCTs, so meta-analysis was not feasible for this outcome, while the SF-36 and MPQ were only reported by single studies. This shows that there is a knowledge gap in terms of the outcome measures used in Chinese medicine clinical research on CR.

In summary, there is some evidence supporting the use of CHM for the management of CR, in particular when oral CHM or topical CHM is used as an add-on therapy to routine care.

References

1. Zhu L, Gao J, Yu J, *et al.* (2015) Jingtong granule: A Chinese patent medicine for cervical spondylotic radiculopathy. *Evid Based Complement Alternat Med* **2015:** 158453.

2. Lee JW, Hyun MK. (2018) Herbal medicine (*Gegen*-decoction) for treating cervical spondylosis: A systematic review and meta-analysis of randomized controlled trials. *Eur J Integr Med* **18**: 52–58.
3. 张鸿升, 周宾宾, 谢忠文, *et al.* (2013) 颈复康颗粒治疗神经根型颈椎病的系统评价. *中西医结合研究* **5**(03): 128–132.
4. 陈超云, 陈培红, 陈斌, *et al.* (2018) 黄芪桂枝五物汤治疗神经根型颈椎病的系统评价. *风湿病与关节炎* **7**(02): 37–42.

References to Included Studies

H1   袁刚, 李峥. (2017) 痹祺胶囊对神经根型颈椎病初次发作神经症状的影响. *中华中医药杂志* **32**(10): 4756–4758.

H2   陈绍华, 朱伟民, 樊远志. (2012) 葛根黄芪汤加减治疗神经根型颈椎病疗效观察. *中国中医骨伤科杂志* **20**(11): 18–19.

H3   吴萍, 张斌. (2013) 葛根汤合颈椎牵引治疗神经根型颈椎病 83 例. *湖南中医杂志* **29**(1): 69–70.

H4   魏纪湖. (2017) 根痛饮膏方治疗神经根型颈椎病的临床观察 (Thesis). 广西中医药大学.

H5   丁志清. (2016) 桂枝加葛根汤加味治疗风寒湿型神经根型颈椎病的临床观察 (Thesis). 成都中医药大学.

H6   徐腾, 王诗忠, 陈水金, *et al.* (2009) 桂枝加葛根汤结合颈椎牵引治疗神经根型颈椎病 68 例随机对照临床研究. *辽宁中医杂志* **36**(12): 2095–2097.

H7   仲跻申, 张立, 姚宏明. (2015) 桂枝加葛根汤配合牵引治疗神经根型颈椎病临床观察. *风湿病与关节炎* **4**(10): 21–23.

H8   唐国皓, 陈波涛, 冉超, *et al.* (2017) 黄芪通络汤治疗神经根型颈椎病对疼痛麻木的影响. *实用中医药杂志* **33**(8): 898–899.

H9   王海荣, 曹林忠. (2018) 活血化瘀汤联合颈椎牵引治疗神经根型颈椎病临床观察. *新中医* **50**(10): 110–113.

H10 莫敏敏, 花宇琪, 赵凯. (2016) 颈肩痛汤加减治疗神经根型颈椎病 25 例. *陕西中医药大学学报* **39**(4): 62–64.

H11 程平平. (2015) 颈痛颗粒配合牵引疗法治疗神经根型颈椎病的临床疗效观察 (Thesis). 河南中医药大学.

H12 黄晋. (2014) 芪麝丸治疗神经根型颈椎病随机双盲安慰剂对照研究 (Thesis). 甘肃中医学院.

H13 邹天强, 齐润文, 朱明双. (2013) 身痛逐瘀汤合芍药甘草汤治疗神经根型颈椎病疗效观察. *实用中医药杂志* **29**(5): 338–339.

(Continued)

(*Continued*)

H14　江建春, 吴军豪, 石玲, *et al.* (2017) 石氏痰瘀通络汤治疗神经根型颈椎病的临床观察. *上海中医药杂志* **51**(4): 70–72.

H15　王长宏, 王志刚. (2013) 水蛭逐瘀胶囊合用川葛舒筋丸治疗神经根型颈椎病 50 例. *中医研究* **26**(11): 34–35.

H16　孙玉明. (2015) 搜风通络汤治疗神经根型颈椎病 27 例. *河南中医* **35**(10): 2423–2424.

H17　邹震, 郭喜庚. (2017) 藤黄健骨片治疗神经根型颈椎病 64 例临床观察. *湖南中医杂志* **33**(1): 67–68.

H18　秦晴, 王东. (2016) 温经通痹汤治疗神经根型颈椎病风寒阻络证 55 例临床研究. *四川中医* **34**(5): 105–107.

H19　于世超. (2017) 项痹舒筋汤结合牵引治疗气滞血瘀型神经根型颈椎病的临床研究 (Thesis). 河南中医药大学.

H20　史先知, 李其富, 赵振强, *et al.* (2014) 乙哌立松与根痛平颗粒治疗神经根型颈椎病的疗效观察. *中医临床研究* **6**(35): 21–23.

H21　陈孟交, 肖四旺. (2018) 中西医结合治疗神经根型颈椎病42例临床观察. *湖南中医杂志* **34**(5): 85–86.

H22　程建, 马勇, 袁涛. (2013) 中药结合牵引治疗中老年神经根型颈椎病. *中国实验方剂学杂志* **19**(8): 344–346.

H23　李全, 李福安, 卢坚. (2007) 马钱子药膏改善颈椎病患者周围神经压迫症状: 随机对照 306 例效果观察. *中国组织工程研究与临床康复* **11**(23): 4531–4533.

H24　黄睿, 秦鹏俊, 郗姗姗, *et al.* (2016) 通络止痛方外敷配合牵引治疗神经根型颈椎病疗效观察. *亚太传统医药* **12**(7): 148–149.

H25　王力平, 梁冬波, 黄承军, *et al.* (2012) 药盐熨烫法治疗神经根型颈椎病疗效观察. *现代中西医结合杂志* **21**(31): 3440–3441.

H26　王玥. (2013) 药熨法治疗神经根型颈椎病气滞血瘀证的临床疗效观察 (Thesis). 湖南中医药大学.

H27　刘浪琪. (2008) 中药离子导入法治疗神经根型颈椎病临床研究 (Thesis). 广州中医药大学.

H28　钱雪华, 孙鹏, 毕联阳, *et al.* (2006) 中药离子导入配合牵引治疗神经根型颈椎病 60 例. *上海中医药杂志* **40**(7): 47–48.

H29　张伟. (2011) 中药热敷疗法治疗颈椎病神经根型的临床研究 (Thesis). 长春中医药大学.

H30　赵歆昱. (2011) 臂痛灵治疗神经根型颈椎病 30 例临床观察. *河北中医* **33**(6): 846.

(*Continued*)

H31 赵建, 崔书国, 国延军, *et al.* (2005) 补肾壮骨活血汤配合中药熏蒸治疗神经根型颈椎病 589 例. *河北中医药学报* **20**(2): 12,4.

H32 李忠伟. (2010) 葛根汤加减治疗神经根型颈椎病 40 例. *江苏中医药* **42**(10): 41.

H33 王龙, 张红星, 邹燃, *et al.* (2014) 根痛合剂治疗神经根型颈椎病 100 例. *光明中医* **29**(9): 1856–1858.

H34 王来群, 辛丽, 孙凤敏. (2008) 骨康散治疗神经根型颈椎病 62 例. *河南中医* **28**(9): 60–61.

H35 王元德, 张庆和. (1999) 黄芪桂枝五物汤加味治疗神经根型颈椎病 60 例. *黑龙江中医药* **02**: 40.

H36 叶秀兰, 李晓锋, 李军. (2012) 筋痹方治疗神经根型颈椎病 150 例临床观察. *上海中医药杂志* **46**(5): 58–60.

H37 路绪文, 赵坤. (2000) 颈痹灵药酒治疗颈椎病疗效观察. *时珍国医国药* **11**(12): 1115.

H38 万全增, 段斌斌, 汪煌, *et al.* (2011) 颈脉通内服配合中药薰蒸治疗神经根型颈椎病 86 例. *中医正骨* **23**(6): 60,3.

H39 张锡智, 刘云涛. (2008) 颈痛颗粒治疗神经根型颈椎病 43 例. *实用中医内科杂志* **22**(2): 69–70.

H40 董博, 袁普卫, 姚洁, *et al.* (2013) 颈痛消胶囊治疗神经根型颈椎病 120 例. *中国中医骨伤科杂志* **21**(3): 49–50.

H41 陈迪光. (2016) 颈椎病经方治验三则. *湖北中医杂志* **38**(11): 52–53.

H42 徐华, 马俊明, 叶洁, *et al.* (2014) 鹿灵活络合剂治疗神经根型颈椎病疗效观察. *辽宁中医杂志* **41**(10): 2149–2151.

H43 陈熙凡, 许敬人. (2001) 祛风活血法治疗神经根性颈椎病及其对血液流变学的影响. *医学理论与实践* **14**(7): 641–642.

H44 江建春, 邱德华, 王敖明, *et al.* (2013) 石氏方药内服外敷治疗神经根型颈椎病 120 例. *中医正骨* **25**(11): 53–55.

H45 梁德, 崔健超, 张华健, *et al.* (2016) 舒筋通络颗粒治疗神经根型和椎动脉型颈椎病 2170 例临床观察. *中医杂志* **57**(14): 1226–1230.

H46 周瑞堂, 贾福奎. (2006) 外用结合内服中药治疗神经根型颈椎病 176 例. *中医外治杂志* **15**(2): 30–31.

H47 朱巨锦. (2010) 应用施杞教授筋痹方治疗神经根型颈椎病 32 例临床体会. *中国社区医师·医学专业* **12**(21): 160.

H48 王力平, 梁冬波, 黄承军, *et al.* (2012) 药盐熨烫法治疗神经根型颈椎病 50 例临床分析. *颈腰痛杂志* **33**(2): 151–152.

6

Pharmacological Actions of Frequently Used Herbs

OVERVIEW

The therapeutic effects of herbal medicine are largely attributable to their active compounds. This chapter provides a summary of experimental evidence of the possible biological activities and mechanisms of the ten most frequently used Chinese herbs from randomised clinical trials discussed in Chapter 5.

Introduction

As mentioned in Chapter 5, a number of systematic reviews have evaluated the potential effects of Chinese herbal medicine (CHM) for cervical radiculopathy (CR) with some promising results found. The evidence from clinical studies included in Chapter 5 has also shown benefits of CHM in alleviating CR symptoms. If such treatments are playing a role in the clinical management of CR, it is important to examine how CHMs exert their clinical effects. This chapter reviews experimental evidence from *in vitro* experimental cells and *in vivo* animal models for some of the most frequently used herbs in clinical trials.

The pathological processes and mechanisms of CR have been described in Chapter 1. Cervical intervertebral disc degeneration, spinal cord compression/injury (SCC/SCI) and neuroinflammation are the key factors contributing to the progression of CR, which is characterised by pain and numbness of the neck and arm.

The following ten herbs and one formula were reviewed: *ge gen* 葛根, *shao yao* 芍药, *huang qi* 黄芪, *gui zhi* 桂枝, *chuan xiong* 川芎, *dang gui* 当归, *gan cao* 甘草, *hong hua* 红花, *qiang huo* 羌活, *ji xue teng* 鸡血藤 and *gen tong ping ke li* (granule) 根痛平颗粒.

Methods

To identify experimental studies in relation to their pharmacological actions of relevance to CR, the activities of each herb and/or main compounds were examined to identify their therapeutic effects on attenuating neuroinflammation (such as in microglial cells and astrocytes *in vitro* and neuron-related inflammatory animals), protecting neurons from damage, injury and degeneration (such as neuroprotection and anti-apoptosis) and relieving pain and/or achieving muscle relaxation (such as neuropathic pain, inflammatory pain and muscle spasms).

The constituent compounds were identified by searching herbal monographs, high-quality reviews of CHM, materia medica and PubMed.[1,2] To identify pre-clinical studies, a literature search in PubMed, Google Scholar and PubMed Central was undertaken. Search terms included the scientific names of the plant, as well as the Chinese *pinyin*, and the names of the main compounds found in the plants. These were combined with terms for CR, neuroinflammation, neuro-oxidative stress, neuroprotection, neuro-apoptosis, analgesia, neuropathic pain, myorelaxation and SCC/SCI rodent models.

Experimental Studies of Herbal Formulae

Gen tong ping ke li (granules) 根痛平颗粒 (GTP), widely used in treating CR, contain most of the common herbs used in clinical studies, such as Radix *Paeoniae*, Radix *Puerariae*, *Carthamus tinctorius*, and so forth, and demonstrated its neuroprotective activity in a rat model of CR induced by SCC/SCI.[3] GTP granules improved motor function recovery and somatosensory-evoked potentials such as amelioration of gait and amplitude, and decreased neuropathic pain after SCC/SCI by inhibiting the expression of tumour necrosis factor-α

(TNF-α) and Bax, and enhancing the expressions of B-cell lymphoma 2 (Bcl-2), neurofilament 200 (NF200) and neuron regeneration through the activation of peroxisome proliferator-activated receptor gamma (PPAR-γ) in the spinal cord tissues.[3]

Experimental Studies of *ge gen* 葛根

Ge gen 葛根 (Radix *Puerariae*), the dried root of *Pueraria lobata* (Wild.) Ohwi belonging to the family Fabaceae or Leguminosae, has been traditionally used for treatment of cardiovascular diseases, cerebrovascular disorders, cancer, diabetes and diabetic complications. Over 70 chemical constituents of Radix *Puerariae* have been identified, including isoflavones, isoflavone glycosides, coumarins, puerarols, oleanenetype triterpenes and triterpenoid glycosides. Among the isolated isoflavone constituents, puerarin, daidzin and daidzein are the three most abundant components.[4] These compounds and their derivatives have various pharmacological activities, including anti-inflammatory, antioxidant, anti-Parkinson's disease, anti-Alzheimer's disease, and anti-osteoporotic activities.[4] Pharmacological effects in relation to CR are discussed next.

Anti-Neuroinflammatory and Antioxidant Actions

Neuroinflammation and oxidative stress have been closely associated with neurodegenerative diseases such as Alzheimer's disease, Parkinson's disease, CR, etc. Microglial cells are resident macrophages of the central nervous system. Activation of microglia and subsequent release of neurotoxic factors such as nitric oxide (NO), prostaglandin E2 (PGE2), cyclooxygenase-2 (COX-2) and inflammatory mediators, including TNF-α, interleukin-1β (IL-1β) and IL-6, contribute to neuroinflammation.[5]

Anti-neuroinflammatory and antioxidant actions of Radix *Puerariae* may be attributed to its various bioactive compounds. Puerarin has attracted a lot of attention due to its high content. Total isoflavones from *P. lobata*, which contains the unique isoflavone puerarin, exhibit strong anti-neuroinflammatory activity *in vivo*. It was demonstrated to inhibit astrocytes and microglia activation, and COX-2 upregulation caused by neuronal cell death in the rat hippocampal CA1 region.[6] In addition, the preventive property of puerarin against oxidative stress-induced neurodegeneration was reported in mitochondrial transgenic neuronal cell cybrid models of sporadic Alzheimer's disease. Puerarin acted as a scavenger of intracellular reactive oxygen species (ROS) to protect neurons against apoptosis stimulated by oxidative stress by reducing the Bax/Bcl-2 ratio.[7] *In vitro*, puerarin was also demonstrated to attenuate beta-amyloid (Aβ)-induced oxidative stress in neuronal cultures from the rat hippocampus by scavenging ROS and inhibiting lipid peroxidation via the GSK-3β/ nuclear factor erythroid 2 p45-related factor 2 (Nrf2) signalling pathway.[8]

Neuroprotective and Anti-Apoptosis Actions

A great number of *in vitro* and/or *in vivo* studies have demonstrated that Radix *Puerariae* and its compounds possess strong neuroprotective and anti-apoptosis qualities.[4,9] *In vitro*, phenolic compounds such as genistein, biochanin A and puerarin of *P. lobata* exhibited potent neuroprotective effects by inhibiting Aβ-induced neurotoxicity through inhibiting apoptosis in PC12 cells.[10] This neuroprotective effect was also observed in 1-methyl-4-phenylpyridinium iodide (MPP$^+$)-induced toxicity of PC12 cells and MPP$^+$-induced human neuroblastoma SH-SY5Y cells through reducing cysteinyl aspartate specific proteinase-3 (caspase-3)-like activation.[11,12] *In vivo*, puerarin protected dopaminergic neurons against 6-hydroxydopamine-induced neurotoxicity through inhibition of apoptosis and upregulation of glial cell line-derived neurotrophic factor expression in rats with Parkinson's disease.[12] It was also shown that puerarin protected mouse neurons from Aβ-induced neuronal death by recovering the levels of brain-derived neurotrophic factor (BDNF) and malondialdehyde (MDA) in the hippocampus and cerebral cortex.[13]

More importantly, several studies have shown the therapeutic effect of puerarin in spinal cord injury (SCI) models. Administration of puerarin significantly improved motor function through reversing the decreases in thioredoxin-1 and thioredoxin-2 expression after SCI,[14] decreasing glutamate release and inhibiting metabotropic glutamate receptors' mRNA expression,[15] and depressing the upregulation of p25 and suppressing the downregulation of p35 by way of a roscovitine-like function.[16]

Analgesic/Myorelaxant Actions

Puerarin was reported to significantly reduce neuropathic pain with improvement in the thresholds of mechanical allodynia and thermal hyperalgesia in superficial back-burnt rats[17] and in chronic constriction injury (CCI) model rats[18] mediated by P2X3 receptors in dorsal root ganglion (DRG) neurons. More recently, puerarin demonstrated its analgesic effect on a neuropathic pain animal model created by partial sciatic nerve ligation through suppressing vanilloid-1 and ankyrin-1 in the DRG of rats with neuropathic pain.[19]

In addition to puerarin, daidzin, daidzein, dihydrodaidzein and p-ethylphenol also showed analgesic activities as assessed by the acetic acid-induced writhing test. Additionally, p-ethylphenol showed muscle relaxant activity in the rotarod and horizontal wire test.[20]

Experimental Studies of *shao yao* 芍药

Shao yao 芍药 (Peony/Paeoniae Radix, *Paeoniae*) includes *bai shao* 白芍 (white peony root/*Radix Paeoniae Alba* sourced from *Paeonia lactiflora* Pall) and *chi chao* 赤芍 (red peony root/*Radix Paeoniae Rubra* sourced from *Paeonia lactiflora* Pall or *Paeonia veitchii* Lynch) based on the colour of their roots.[21,22] Monoterpene glycosides, polyphenols and paeonols are the three main types of compounds of Paeoniae Radix. Paeoniflorin is the most abundant and accounts for the pharmacological activity. These compounds have been shown to be multi-functional with anti-inflammatory, antioxidant, anti-arthritis, anti-coagulant and anti-platelet activity, and immunomodulatory activity.[21,22] Pharmacological effects in relation to CR are discussed next.

Anti-Neuroinflammatory and Antioxidant Actions

Paeoniflorin significantly blocked lipopolysaccharide (LPS)-induced hippocampal cell death and production of NO and IL-1β in hippocampal slice cultures and in microglia.[23] It inhibited morphine-induced robust microglial activation by suppressing increases in nuclear factor-κB (NF-κB) translocation and pro-inflammatory cytokine expression, and toll-like receptor-4 (TLR-4) in both microglia and the spinal cord of rats.[24] Furthermore, in interferon-alpha (IFN-α)-induced neuroinflammation, paeoniflorin reversed abnormal levels of IL-6, IL-1β, IL-9, IL-10, IL-12 and TNF-α by influencing the activation of microglia or astrocytes.[25] In addition to paeoniflorin, paeonol was also shown to ameliorate microglia-mediated neuroinflammation and oxidative stress-induced neurotoxicity in rat primary microglial and cortical neurons.[26]

Neuroprotective and Anti-Apoptosis Actions

In rat cortical cells, two monoterpenes — paeonilactone-C and benzoylpaeoniflorin — significantly protected the primary cultures of rat cortical cells against hydrogen peroxide (H_2O_2)-induced neurotoxicity.[27] In primary-cultured hippocampal neurons, paeoniflorin protected neuron cells from N-methyl-D-asparate (NMDA)-induced excitotoxicity via modulation of the Ca^{2+}/calmodulin-dependent protein kinase II (CaMKII)/cyclic adenosine monophosphate (cAMP)-response element binding (CREB) protein signalling pathways.[28] In cerebral injury rat models, paeonol and paeoniflorin showed neuroprotective effects by scavenging superoxide anions, suppressing microglial activation, inhibiting the expression of IL-1β, NFκB and TNF-α,[29] and regulating the CaMKII /CREB signalling pathways.[28]

Analgesic/Myorelaxant Actions

Paeoniflorin has been attracting attention for its anti-nociceptive activities. Paeoniflorin demonstrated dose-related anti-nociception mediated by the activation of kappa-opioid receptors[30] and by an interaction with NMDA receptors.[31] More recently, paeoniflorin was reported to mimic the ASK1 inhibitor NQDI1 to attenuate neuropathic pain in CCI rats by reducing the expressions of p38 and p-JNK.[32] In addition to paeoniflorin, albiflorin also showed antinociceptive activity by reducing the activation of CaMKII and c-JNK in the hypothalamus in Albiflorin-treated mice.[33]

Experimental Studies of *huang qi* 黄芪

Huang qi 黄芪 (*Astragali RadiSx*), belonging to the Leguminosae family, is sourced from the dried roots of *Astragalus membranaceus* and *Astragalus membranaceus var. mongholicus*. More than 200 compounds have been identified including saponins, flavonoids, polysaccharides and amino acids. Among these, the triterpenoid saponin astragaloside IV (AST-IV) is the principal active component of the herb. Crude extracts of *Astragali RadiSx* and constituents have multiple pharmacological effects, including anti-inflammatory, anti-oxidative, anti-fibrotic, and immunostimulant effects.[34] Other pharmacological effects in relation to CR are discussed next.

Anti-Neuroinflammatory and Antioxidant Actions

In vitro, an anti-neuroinflammatory effect of AST-IV was demonstrated in suppressing LPS-induced microglial activation as shown by inhibiting the production of NO, TNF-α and IL-6 in LPS-stimulated microglia and LPS-induced primary microglia isolated from C57BL/6 mice.[35] It was also shown to decrease oxidative stress by eliminating intracellular ROS in SH-SY5Y cells and iNOS expression in microglia.[36] Interestingly, a study of AST-IV on the M1/M2 microglial activation in response to LPS stimulation demonstrated that AST-IV could shift microglia from inflammatory M1 to an anti-inflammatory M2 phenotype.[37] *In vivo*, AST-IV alleviated neuroinflammation by inhibiting astrocytes and microglial activation in mice with chronic neuroinflammation through counteracting oxidative stress.[36] The mechanism of AST-IV in inhibiting neuroinflammation was further explored through modulating glucocorticoid receptor-mediated signalling pathways.[38]

Neuroprotective and Anti-Apoptosis Actions

Numerous studies have demonstrated the neuroprotective effect of *Astragali RadiSx*. Several studies have shown a therapeutic effect of *Astragali RadiSx* on rat SCI due to both its antioxidant and neuroprotective effects. Intraperitoneal injection of *Astragali RadiSx* significantly increased the downregulation of superoxide dismutase (SOD) and decreased MDA expression in the injured spinal cord of SCI rats.[39] It also improved motor function recovery and somatosensory-evoked potentials such as amelioration of gait and amplitude.[40]

In vitro, AST-IV exerted significant neuroprotective activity against oxygen- and glucose deprivation/re-oxygenation (OGD/R)-induced damage in murine cortical neurons by reducing ROS accumulation through activating epidermal growth factor receptor (EGFR)-Nrf2 signalling pathways[41] and protein kinase A (PKA)/CREB pathways.[42] AST-IV ameliorated the H_2O_2-induced apoptosis of neuronal cells in SH-SY5Y cells and glutamate-induced neurotoxicity in PC12 cells to exert protective effects against neurodegeneration through the p38 MAPK pathway[43] and Raf-MEK-ERK pathway,[44] respectively. Furthermore, a microglia-conditioned medium treated with AST-IV promoted PC12 neuron survival and attenuated microglia-mediated neuronal damage compared to an LPS-stimulated BV-2 microglial medium.[37] *In vivo* experiments also showed that AST-IV could reduce the damage and apoptosis of hippocampal neurons and promote the survival of neurons in the cerebral cortex and the growth of axons in mice.[36]

In addition to AST-IV, calycosin, a major isoflavonoid of *Astragali RadiSx*, was demonstrated in *in vitro* primary-cultured neurons and *in vivo* cerebral injury rats to induce neuroprotection by upregulating SOD activity and the antioxidant enzyme glutathione peroxidase (GSH-Px)[45] via the transient receptor potential canonical 6 (TRPC6)/CREB pathway.[46]

Moreover, *A. membranaceus* polysaccharides also demonstrated neuroprotective activity by inhibiting polyglutamine-mediated proteotoxicity through the DAF-16/FOXO transcription factor.[47]

Analgesic/Myorelaxant Actions

An extract of *Astragalus* hydroalcoholic was shown to significantly reduce both sodium monoiodoacetate-induced pain and complete Freund's adjuvant (CFA)-induced pain through inhibiting the release of pro-inflammatory cytokines.[48] A relaxant effect of calycosin on isolated rat thoracic aorta rings pre-contracted with phenylephrine or KCl indicated that calycosin is a non-competitive Ca (2+) channel blocker that may relieve muscle cramps.[49] Kaempferol, another isoflavonoid in *Astragali RadiSx*, was also shown to have a relaxant effect on KCl-induced tonic contractions in isolated rat uteri by modulating the cAMP expression.[50]

Experimental Studies of *gui zhi* 桂枝

Gui zhi 桂枝 (Cinnamon, *Cinnamomum cassia* Presl), belonging to the Lauraceae family, primarily contains essential oils including cinnamaldehyde or cinnamic aldehyde, eugenol and linalool, a variety of resinous derivatives including cinnamaldehyde, cinnamic acid and cinnamate, and numerous other components such as polyphenols with antioxidant, anti-inflammatory, anti-hyperlipidemic, anti-diabetic, anti-microbial, anti-cancer and other beneficial effects against polycystic ovary syndrome, gastric emptying and Parkinson's and Alzheimer's diseases.[51] Other pharmacological effects in relation to CR are discussed next.

Anti-Neuroinflammatory and Antioxidant Actions

A *C. cassia* extract and its main constituent, trans-cinnamaldehyde (TCA), have been shown to significantly inhibit neuroinflammation by reducing the production of NO, IL-1β, IL-6 and TNF-α through blocking NF-κB activation in LPS-stimulated microglia.[52] In a microglial and PC12 cell co-culture system with LPS stimulation, TCA protected neuroinflammation-mediated neuronal damage by blocking the NF-κB signalling pathway.[53] *In vivo*, TCA improved memory deficits and synaptic plasticity inhibition in the hippocampus by suppressing microglial activation and neuroinflammation in LPS-challenged mice.[54] In the mouse hippocampus and prefrontal cortex, TCA diminished microglial activation and pro-inflammatory mediators by blocking the NF-κB signalling pathway.[55]

In addition to TCA, 2'-Hydroxycinnamaldehyde (HCA) and its derivative 2'-benzoyloxycinnamaldehyde (BCA) also showed a potential anti-neuroinflammatory effect in LPS-stimulated microglial cultures and microglia/neuroblastoma co-cultures by targeting the low-density lipoprotein receptor-related protein 1 (LRP1).[56]

Neuroprotective and Anti-Apoptosis Actions

A cinnamon extract markedly inhibited the formation of toxic Aβ oligomers and prevented Aβ-mediated cytotoxicity in rat neuronal PC12 cells.[57] The total flavonoids of cinnamon were found to protect PC12 cells from 6-hydroxydopamine injury, enhance the activity of SOD, alleviate DNA damage and decrease the expression levels of the Bax/Bcl-2 ratio.[58] *In vivo*, cinnamon extract recovered the locomotion defects and totally eliminated the tetrameric species of Aβ in the brain in a fly model of Alzheimer's disease.[57] TCA treatment exhibited potent neuroprotective effects as shown by ameliorating cognition decline, abnormal expression of synaptic proteins and NMDA receptor (NMDAR) dysfunction in PS cDKO mice.[55]

Analgesic/Myorelaxant Actions

A *C. cassia* extract was reported to have an effective analgesic effect on oxaliplatin-induced neuropathic pain as demonstrated by a potent anti-allodynic effect via inhibiting the activation of astrocytes and microglia, and decreasing the expression of IL-1β and TNF α in the spinal cord after an injection with oxaliplatin.[59] More recently, cinnamic acid was reported to provide relief from neuropathic pain against oxaliplatin-induced cold and mechanical hypersensitivity in rats through inhibiting spinal pain transmission.[60] In addition, an anti-nociceptive effect of essential oils from *C. cassia* was shown in models of acetic acid-induced writhing, oxytocin-induced writhing, formalin- and CFA-induced overt pain tests and carrageenan-stimulated mechanical hyperalgesia through suppressing inflammatory activity.[61]

Experimental Studies of *chuan xiong* 川芎

Chuan xiong 川芎 (*Ligusticum chuanxiong* Hort), belonging to the Umbelliferae family, is used for the treatment of migraine and various cardiovascular and cerebrovascular diseases. So far more than 200 compounds have been isolated and identified from *L. chuanxiong* and these can be grouped into five basic types: volatile oil, phenols and organic acids, alkaloids, phthalides and polysaccharides. Ferulic acid (FA), ligustilide, tetramethylpyrazine (TMP, also known as ligustrazine) and senkyunolide A are the main active constituents of *L. chuanxiong*.[62] These compounds demonstrate a broad therapeutic capacity, including effects on antioxidation, anti-inflammation, and so forth.[62] Pharmacological effects in relation to CR are discussed next.

Anti-Neuroinflammatory and Antioxidant Actions

Senkyunolide A and *Z*-ligustilide were found to inhibit the production of pro-inflammatory mediators in LPS-stimulated microglia. Both compounds could protect neuro-2a cells from neuroinflammatory toxicity induced by LPS-stimulated microglial culture media.[63] More recently, senkyunolide H further demonstrated attenuation of MPP+-induced neurotoxicity, oxidative stress and apoptosis in PC12 cells.[64]

In addition, TMP not only inhibited Aβ25–35 and interferon-γ (IFN-γ)-stimulated production of NO, TNF-α, IL-1β, ROS and NF-κB activation in cultured microglia, but also blocked Aβ25–35-induced ROS generation in organotypic hippocampal slice cultures.[65] FA was reported to blunt rat ischemic detrimental brain injury by acting as a hydroxyl radical scavenger and via anti-inflammatory activity.[66] Moreover, butylidenephthalide from *L. chuanxiong* was reported to inhibit LPS-induced production of NO, TNF-α and IL-1β by repressing microglial activation in rat brain microglia and in organotypic hippocampal slice cultures.[67]

Neuroprotective and Anti-Apoptosis Actions

The protective effects of ligustilide and TMP against neural damage have been extensively studied in recent years with multiple mechanisms. Ligustilide demonstrated a protective effect against I/R-induced damage to the rat brain *in vivo* and rat-cultured neurons *in vitro* by promoting erythropoietin (EPO) transcription and inhibiting a stress-induced protein RTP801 expression.[68] Using a glioma-neuronal co-culturing system, TMP was shown to effectively inhibit glioma cells and protect primary-cultured cerebral neurocytes against H_2O_2-induced damage by downregulating the chemokine receptor CXCR4 expression.[69] TMP neuroprotection against kainate-induced excitotoxicity was through quenching of ROS and reducing of intracellular calcium, and inhibiting of glutamate-induced neuronal death *in vivo* and *in vitro*.[70] TMP effectively prevented a 1-methyl-4-phenyl-1,2,3,6-tetrahydropyridine (MPTP)-induced dopaminergic neuron injury in a rat model of Parkinson's disease by preventing the downregulation of Nrf2 and glutamate-cysteine ligase catalytic subunit (GCLc), maintaining redox balance and inhibiting apoptosis.[71] In SCI rats, TMP improved rat motor functions and protected the injured spinal cord by suppressing inflammatory cytokines, inhibiting cell apoptosis and scavenging oxygen free radicals.[72]

Analgesic/Myorelaxant Actions

TMP showed anti-nociceptive effects with elevation of the threshold of thermal nociception and prolongation of the withdrawal latency of ipsilateral hindpaw to noxious heating by inhibiting the high-voltage gated calcium current and tetrodotoxin-resistant sodium current of DRG neurons in rats.[73] More recently, TMP was reported to significantly improve CCI-induced neuroinflammatory and neuro-pathic pain by suppressing the expression of MMP-2 and MMP-9 and the phosphorylation of JNK via the TAK1 signalling pathway in astrocytes.[74]

In addition, the volatile oil was also reported to improve the mouse hot plate-induced pain threshold and reduce the acetic acid-induced writhing reaction accompanied with decreases in the expression of c-fos and the secretion of calcitonin gene-related peptides in brain tissue and an increase in the content of 5-hydroxytryptamine in plasma.[75]

Ligustilide was reported to have a centrally acting muscle-relaxant effect on the crossed extensor reflex in anesthetised rats.[76] *Z*-ligustilide had an anti-spasmodic effect on the ileum, colon and vas deferens of guinea pigs and antagonised contractions of the uterus.[77]

Experimental Studies of *dang gui* 当归

Dang gui 当归 (*Radix Angelica Sinensis*) consists of over 70 compounds. FA, *Z*-ligustilide, butylidenephthalide, butylphthalide and polysaccharide are thought to be the main active components in *A. sinensis.* These compounds have diverse biological activities, including anti-inflammatory, antioxidant, anti-arthrosclerosis, and immuno-modulatory activity.[78] Pharmacological effects in relation to CR are discussed next.

Anti-Neuroinflammatory and Antioxidant Actions

Pre-treatment with angelica polysaccharide was reported to alleviate LPS-induced inflammation and apoptosis in rat pheochromocytoma PC12 neuron cells by reducing the expression levels of IL-1β, IL-6, IL-8, TNF-α and COX-1 through the PI3K/AKT pathway.[79]

Neuroprotective and Anti-Apoptosis Actions

Z-ligustilide exerted a pronounced neuroprotective effect against H_2O_2-induced cytotoxicity in PC12 cells through improving antioxidant defence and inhibiting mitochondrial apotosis.[80] *In vivo*, Z-ligustilide treatment could protect brain injury by increasing the activities of GSH-PX, SOD and anti-apoptosis in ICR mouse ischemic brain tissues.[81] This finding was extended and confirmed in ligustilide by involving inhibition of TLR4/peroxiredoxin 6 signalling.[82]

Analgesic/Myorelaxant Actions

A water extract of *A. Sinensis* possessed significant analgesic activity by decreasing the acetic acid-induced frequency of the wringing reaction and increasing the pain threshold in a hot-plate procedure in mice.[83] Sodium ferulate blocked the initiation of pain and primary afferent sensitisation in CCI rats.[84] Moreover, FA reversed reserpine-induced decreases in the nociceptive threshold in both thermal hyperalgesia and mechanical allodynia by modulating the monoaminergic system.[85] The study was further extended to CCI-induced neuropathic pain by the same research group.[86]

Additionally, ligustilide, butylidenephthalide and butylphthalide were found to be capable of relaxing rat uterine contractions and other smooth muscle systems as non-specific antispasmodics.[87]

Experimental Studies of *gan cao* 甘草

Gan cao 甘草 (licorice) from *Glycyrrhiza uralensis* Fisch., *Glycyrrhiza inflata* Bat. and *Glycyrrhiza glabra* L has been traditionally used to treat coughs, influenza, gastric ulcers and liver damage and detoxification. Among at least 400 isolated compounds, the main bioactive constituents of licorice are triterpene saponins (more than 20) and various types of flavonoids (more than 300). These compounds exhibit extensive pharmacological properties such as anti-inflammatory, anti-allergic, antioxidative, and immunoregulatory effects.[88] Pharmacological effects in relation to CR are discussed next.

Anti-Neuroinflammatory and Antioxidant Actions

Glabridin, a flavonoid isolated from *G. glabra*, was reported to inhibit microglial activation by blocking the DNA-binding activity of NF-κB and AP-1.[89] Glycyrrhizin, a triterpenoid saponin from *G. glabra*, demonstrated anti-neuroinflammatory activity in systemic LPS-treated mice through inhibiting pro-inflammatory cytokines and ionised calcium-binding adaptor molecule 1 (Iba1, a marker of microglial activation in the hippocampal tissue).[90] Additionally, glycyrrhizic acid, liquiritin and liquiritigenin also demonstrated anti-neuroinflammatory activities in microglial cells.[91] More recently, glycyrrhizic acid was confirmed to work against LPS-induced neuroinflammation in an LPS-induced Alzheimer's mouse model through inhibiting activation of the TLR4 signalling pathway.[92]

Neuroprotective and Anti-Apoptosis Actions

The neuroprotective activity of licorice has been largely attributed to an active component, isoliquiritigenin (ISL), a flavonoid from *G. glabra*. It has been shown that ISL protected HT22 hippocampal neuronal cells from glutamate-induced mitochondrial damage and cell death through inhibiting the expression of the apoptotic regulators Bcl-2 and Bax, and suppressing glutamate-induced ROS production.[93] It also protected cultured cortical neurons from Aβ (25–35)-induced neuronal apoptosis by interfering with increases in ([Ca^{2+}]$_i$) and ROS.[94] In animal models of cerebral I/R injury, pre-treatment with ISL significantly reduced the cerebral infarct volume and oedema, and produced significant reduction in neurological deficits due to the amelioration of cerebral energy metabolism and its antioxidant property.[95] Another compound, liquiritin from flavonoids, showed a similar neuroprotective effect through antioxidant and anti-apoptosis properties.[96]

Analgesic/Myorelaxant Actions

ISL not only demonstrated analgesic and uterine relaxant effects *in vitro*, but also showed effective activity in reducing pain in the acetic acid-induced writhing response and hot-plate test *in vivo* through involvement of Ca^{2+} channels, NOS and COX.[97] Liquiritin was proven to have protective efficacy on CCI-induced neuropathic pain in mice by significantly alleviating CCI-evoked behavioural variations in mechanical allodynia, cold allodynia and thermal hyperalgesia. Moreover, the protective effect on CCI-induced neuropathic pain of liquiritin was attributed to its anti-inflammatory actions.[98]

Experimental Studies of *hong hua* 红花

Hong hua 红花 (*Carthamus tinctorius* L.; safflower) contains many chemical constituents, including quinochalcones, flavonoids, alkaloids, polyacetylenes, alkanediol, fatty acids, steroids, lignans, etc. In particular, quinochalcone C-glycoside hydroxysafflor yellow A (HSYA), N-(p-Coumaroyl) serotonin and N-feruloylserotonin are responsible for most of the pharmacological activities, such as anti-oxidant, anti-osteoporosis and anti-atherosclerosis activities.[99] Pharmacological effects in relation to CR are discussed next.

Anti-Neuroinflammatory and Antioxidant Actions

The major component of the yellow pigment HSYA has attracted the most attention and is a promising therapeutic agent for neurodegenerative diseases. *In vitro*, HSYA was demonstrated to suppress $A\beta_{1-42}$-induced neuroinflammation in $A\beta_{1-42}$-treated microglia by reducing the expression of the pro-inflammatory mediators and protecting primary cortical neuronal cells and SH-SY5Y cells against microglia-mediated neurotoxicity through Janus Kinase 2 (JAK2)/signal transducers and activators of the transcription 3 (STAT3) pathway.[100] In LPS-activated microglia, HSYA suppressed LPS-induced TLR4 expression and protected neuronal damage at the early stage of LPS stimulation.[101] Moreover, in primary mesencephalic cultures, HSYA could decrease the content of IL-1β, TNF-α and NO, partially inhibit the expressions of NF-κB p65 and iNOS, and attenuate LPS-induced dopaminergic neuron damage.[102] *In vivo*, HSYA was reported to alleviate MPTP-induced neurotoxicity in a Parkinson's disease mouse model by inhibiting oxidative stress with increases in the activity of SOD, catalase activity and GSH levels, and decreases in MDA and hydroxyl radicals.[103]

Neuroprotective and Anti-Apoptosis Actions

In a primary-cultured rat cortical neuronal model, HSYA showed protective effects on cortical neurons through regulating the Bcl-2 family.[104] As for PC12 cells, HSYA significantly protected these cells from neurotoxicity induced by Aβ as evidenced by reversing the changes triggered by Aβ.[105] *In vivo*, an extract of *C. tinctorius* seeds displayed a neuroprotective effect through antioxidative and anti-inflammatory mechanisms.[106] In particular, HSYA protected spinal cords from I/R injury in rabbits. It not only improved neurological outcomes, but also attenuated I/R-induced necrosis in spinal cords through alleviating oxidative stress and reducing neuronal apoptosis.[107]

In addition to HSYA, N-(p-Coumaroyl) serotonin and N-feruroylserotonin have been reported to possess neuroprotective activity. Treatment with kaempferol-3-O-rutinoside (KRS) and kaempferol-3-O-glucoside (KGS) protected neuron and axon damage after I/R in rats by inhibition of STAT3 and NF-κB activation.[108]

Analgesic/Myorelaxant Actions

The *C. tinctorius* was shown to possess central analgesic activity through proteolytic degradation of tyrosinase, which is responsible for inhibition of the monoaminergic neurotransmitter.[109] Additionally, a hydroalcoholic extract (HE), KRS and KGS also exerted anti-nociceptive effects in mice by significantly reducing both acetic acid-induced and formalin-induced nociceptive responses and cinnamaldehyde-induced paw oedema through suppressing inflammation.[110]

Experimental Studies of *qiang huo* 羌活

Qianghuo 羌活 (*Notopterygium incisum* Ting ex H.T. Chang and *Notopterygium franchetii* H. de Boissieuas), belonging to the family

Apiaceae, has been used to effectively treat the common cold, headache and rheumatism. It contains multiple components including coumarins, steroids, polyacetylenes and essential oils, which exert diaphoretic, analgesic and anti-inflammatory properties.[111] Pharmacological effects in relation to CR are discussed next.

Anti-Neuroinflammatory and Antioxidant Actions

A great number of *in vitro* and/or *in vivo* studies have demonstrated overall/global anti-inflammatory and antioxidant effects of *Notopterygium*, which in turn benefit the head, neck and shoulders.[111] However, specific anti-neuroinflammatory and antioxidant activity has not been reported.

Analgesic/Myorelaxant Actions

An *n*-hexane extract of *N. incisum* was found to inhibit the activities of 5-lipoxygenase and cyclooxygenase (COX), which are associated with analgesic activity *in vitro*. Two major constituents, phen-ethyl ferulate and falcarindiol, were identified to be responsible for the inhibitory effect.[112] *In vivo*, a methanolic extract of *N. incisum* inhibited acetic acid-induced writhing at an inhibition rate of 87% in mice, while an *n*-butanol extract exhibited a strong inhibitory effect. The compound notopterol was identified to have a strong analgesic effect.[113]

Experimental Studies of *ji xue teng* 鸡血藤

Ji xue teng 鸡血藤 (*Spatholobus suberectus* Dunn), belonging to the Leguminosae family, has been traditionally used for the management of anaemia, rheumatism, abnormality in menstruation and other disorders. The vine stem of *S. suberectus* is also well known as Spatholobi Caulis (SC), which contains the major active ingredients, including eriodictyol, dihydroquercetin, butin, neoisoliquiritigenin, plathymenin, dihydrokaempferol and liquiritigenin, which possess various activities such as anti-inflammatory, antioxidant activities.[114] Pharmacological effects in relation to CR are discussed next.

Neuroprotective and Anti-Apoptosis Actions

A neuroprorective effect of an aqueous extract of the stem of *S. suberectus* in cerebral ischemic rats has been demonstrated by decreasing the expressions of TNF-α, caspase 3, NF-κB, MDA and NO, and increasing the expressions of IL-10, ATP and the activity of SOD and GPX in the brain tissues of cerebral ischemic rats through antioxidant, anti-apoptotic and anti-inflammatory activities.[115] Moreover, *in vitro*, SC could protect neuronal cells against etoposide-induced cell viability loss in SH-SY5Y cells by ameliorating apoptotic phenotypes, including poly(ADP-ribose) polymerase, caspase-3 and oxidative stress. *In vivo*, SC could improve neuronal survival and the level of BDNF by suppressing glial activation, oxidative stress and apoptosis in the ipsilateral cortex.[116] Formononetin, an isoflavone from *S. suberectus*, showed a neuroprotective effect against NMDA-invoked neurotoxicity in primary-cultured cortical neurons through inhibiting apoptosis by increasing the levels of Bcl-2 and pro-caspase-3, and decreasing the levels of Bax and caspase-3.[117]

Summary of Pharmacological Actions of the Common Herbs

Each of these 10 herbs has attracted research attention in experimental models of relevance to CR. Overall/global anti-inflammatory and antioxidant effects have been reported in all 10 herbs and have been known to enhance the immune system against whole-body inflammation, which in turn is beneficial to the head, neck and shoulders. Specific anti-neuroinflammatory and antioxidant actions were also observed in most of these herbs with strong effects, except for *dang gui* 当归, *qiang huo* 羌活 and *ji xue teng* 鸡血藤, through suppressing the activation of microglial cells and astrocytes, and subsequently reducing the release of inflammatory mediators and free radicals.

Neuroprotective and anti-apoptosis actions were also observed in most of the herbs. With the exception of *qiang huo* 羌活, all showed powerful neuroprotective properties through suppressing neuroinflammation, oxidant stress and apoptosis.

The actions of relieving pain and/or relaxing muscles were observed in most of the herbs, except for *ji xue teng* 鸡血藤, through suppressing the expression of inflammatory mediators, activating the kappa-opioid receptor, modulating the neurotransmitters in the central nervous system and alleviating nociceptive transmission in DRG.

In addition, most of these herbs have been assessed in SCI or CCI rodent models, except for *gui zhi* 桂枝, *qiang huo* 羌活 and *ji xue teng* 鸡血藤, through anti-inflammatory, antioxidant, neuroprotective or anti-apoptosis effects. However, assessment in CR-specific models was not observed except for one formula, *Gen tong ping ke li* 根痛平颗粒. Further studies with CR models could provide more guidance for the use of CHM in clinical practice.

These *in vitro* and *in vivo* studies examined herb actions specific to CR and provide potential explanations of the clinical benefits of all these common herbs. The findings highlight that CHM herbs have multiple components, which can act on multiple pathways relevant to CR.

References

1. Zhou J, Xie G, Yan X. (2011) *Encyclopedia of Traditional Chinese Medicine: Molecular Structures, Pharmacological Activities, Natural Sources and Applications.* Springer, Berlin, Germany.
2. Bensky D, Clavey S, Stoger E. (2004) *Chinese Herbal Medicine: Materia Medica, 3rd edn.* Eastland Press, Seattle, United States.
3. Sun W, Zheng K, Liu B, *et al.* (2017) Neuroprotective potential of *gentongping* in rat model of cervical spondylotic radiculopathy targeting PPAR-gamma pathway. *J Immunol Res* **2017**: 9152960.
4. Zhang Z, Lam TN, Zuo Z. (2013) Radix puerariae: An overview of its chemistry, pharmacology, pharmacokinetics, and clinical use. *J Clin Pharmacol* **53**(8): 787–811.
5. Lee M. (2013) Neurotransmitters and microglial-mediated neuroinflammation. *Curr Protein Pept Sci* **14**(1): 21–32.

6. Lim DW, Lee C, Kim IH, Kim YT. (2013) Anti-inflammatory effects of total isoflavones from Pueraria lobata on cerebral ischemia in rats. *Molecules* **18**(9): 10404–10412.

7. Zhang H, Liu Y, Lao M, *et al.* (2011) Puerarin protects Alzheimer's disease neuronal cybrids from oxidant-stress-induced apoptosis by inhibiting pro-death signaling pathways. *Exp Gerontol* **46**(1): 30–37.

8. Zou Y, Hong B, Fan L, *et al.* (2013) Protective effect of puerarin against beta-amyloid-induced oxidative stress in neuronal cultures from rat hippocampus: Involvement of the GSK-3β/Nrf2 signaling pathway. *Free Radic Res* **47**(1): 55–63.

9. Zhou YX, Zhang H, Peng C. (2014) Puerarin: A review of pharmacological effects. *Phytother Res* **28**(7): 961–975.

10. Choi YH, Hong SS, Shin YS, *et al.* (2010) Phenolic compounds from *Pueraria lobata* protect PC12 cells against Aβ-induced toxicity. *Arch Pharm Res* **33**(10): 1651–1654.

11. Wang G, Zhou L, Zhang Y, *et al.* (2011) Implication of the c-Jun-NH$_2$-terminal kinase pathway in the neuroprotective effect of puerarin against 1-methyl-4-phenylpyridinium (MPP$^+$)-induced apoptosis in PC-12 cells. *Neurosci Lett* **487**(1): 88–93.

12. Zhu G, Wang X, Wu S, Li Q. (2012) Involvement of activation of PI3K/Akt pathway in the protective effects of puerarin against MPP$^+$-induced human neuroblastoma SH-SY5Y cell death. *Neurochem Int* **60**(4): 400–408.

13. Wu L, Tong T, Wan S, *et al.* (2017) Protective effects of puerarin against abeta 1-42-induced learning and memory impairments in mice. *Planta Med* **83**(3–4): 224–231.

14. Tian F, Xu LH, Zhao W, *et al.* (2011) The optimal therapeutic timing and mechanism of puerarin treatment of spinal cord ischemia–reperfusion injury in rats. *J Ethnopharmacol* **134**(3): 892–896.

15. Tian F, Xu LH, Zhao W, *et al.* (2013) The neuroprotective mechanism of puerarin treatment of acute spinal cord injury in rats. *Neurosci Lett* **543**: 64–68.

16. Tian F, Xu LH, Wang B, *et al.* (2015) The neuroprotective mechanism of puerarin in the treatment of acute spinal ischemia–reperfusion injury is linked to cyclin-dependent kinase 5. *Neurosci Lett* **584**: 50–55.

17. Xu C, Li G, Gao Y, *et al.* (2009) Effect of puerarin on P2X3 receptor involved in hyperalgesia after burn injury in the rat. *Brain Res Bull* **80**(6): 341–346.

18. Xu C, Xu W, Xu H, *et al.* (2012) Role of puerarin in the signalling of neuropathic pain mediated by P2X3 receptor of dorsal root ganglion neurons. *Brain Res Bull* **87**(1): 37–43.

19. Xie HT, Xia ZY, Pan X, *et al.* (2018) Puerarin ameliorates allodynia and hyperalgesia in rats with peripheral nerve injury. *Neural Regen Res* **13**(7): 1263–1268.

20. Yasuda T, Endo M, Kon-no T, *et al.* (2005) Antipyretic, analgesic and muscle relaxant activities of pueraria isoflavonoids and their metabolites from Pueraria lobata Ohwi — A traditional Chinese drug. *Biol Pharm Bull* **28**(7): 1224–1228.

21. Parker S, May B, Zhang C, *et al.* (2016) A pharmacological review of bioactive constituents of Paeonia lactiflora Pallas and Paeonia veitchii Lynch. *Phytother Res* **30**(9): 1445–1473.

22. Yan B, Shen M, Fang J, *et al.* (2018) Advancement in the chemical analysis of Paeoniae Radix (Shaoyao). *J Pharm Biomed Anal* **160**: 276–288.

23. Nam KN, Yae CG, Hong JW, *et al.* (2013) Paeoniflorin, a monoterpene glycoside, attenuates lipopolysaccharide-induced neuronal injury and brain microglial inflammatory response. *Biotechnol Lett* **35**(8): 1183–1189.

24. Jiang C, Xu L, Chen L, *et al.* (2015) Selective suppression of microglial activation by paeoniflorin attenuates morphine tolerance. *Eur J Pain* **19**(7): 908–919.

25. Li J, Huang S, Huang W, *et al.* (2017) Paeoniflorin ameliorates interferon-alpha-induced neuroinflammation and depressive-like behaviors in mice. *Oncotarget* **8**(5): 8264–8282.

26. Tseng YT, Hsu YY, Shih YT, Lo YC. (2012) Paeonol attenuates microglia-mediated inflammation and oxidative stress–induced neurotoxicity in rat primary microglia and cortical neurons. *Shock* **37**(3): 312–318.

27. Kim SH, Lee MK, Lee KY, *et al.* (2009) Chemical constituents isolated from Paeonia lactiflora roots and their neuroprotective activity against oxidative stress in vitro. *J Enzyme Inhib Med Chem* **24**(5): 1138–1140.

28. Zhang Y, Qiao L, Xu W, *et al.* (2017) Paeoniflorin attenuates cerebral ischemia-induced injury by regulating Ca^{2+}/CaMKII/CREB signaling pathway. *Molecules* **22**(3): 359.

29. Tang NY, Liu CH, Hsieh CT, Hsieh CL. (2010) The anti-inflammatory effect of paeoniflorin on cerebral infarction induced by ischemia-reperfusion injury in Sprague-Dawley rats. *Am J Chin Med* **38**(1): 51–64.

30. Tsai HY, Lin YT, Tsai CH, Chen YF. (2001) Effects of paeoniflorin on the formalin-induced nociceptive behaviour in mice. *J Ethnopharmacol* **75**(2–3): 267–271.

31. Chen YF, Lee MM, Fang HL, *et al.* (2016) Paeoniflorin inhibits excitatory amino acid agonist and high-dose morphine-induced nociceptive behavior in mice via modulation of N-methyl-D-aspartate receptors. *BMC Complement Altern Med* **16**: 240.

32. Zhou D, Zhang S, Hu L, *et al.* (2019) Inhibition of apoptosis signal-regulating kinase by paeoniflorin attenuates neuroinflammation and ameliorates neuropathic pain. *J Neuroinflammation* **16**(1): 83.

33. Zhang Y, Sun D, Meng Q, *et al.* (2016) Calcium channels contribute to albiflorin-mediated antinociceptive effects in mouse model. *Neurosci Lett* **628**: 105–109.

34. Fu J, Wang Z, Huang L, *et al.* (2014) Review of the botanical characteristics, phytochemistry, and pharmacology of Astragalus membranaceus (*Huangqi*). *Phytother Res* **28**(9): 1275–1283.

35. Li C, Yang F, Liu F, *et al.* (2018) NRF2/HO-1 activation via ERK pathway involved in the anti-neuroinflammatory effect of Astragaloside IV in LPS-induced microglial cells. *Neurosci Lett* **666**: 104–110.

36. He Y, Du M, Gao Y, *et al.* (2013) Astragaloside IV attenuates experimental autoimmune encephalomyelitis of mice by counteracting oxidative stress at multiple levels. *PLoS One* **8**(10): e76495.

37. Yu J, Guo M, Li Y, *et al.* (2019) Astragaloside IV protects neurons from microglia-mediated cell damage through promoting microglia polarization. *Folia Neuropathol* **57**(2): 170–181.

38. Liu HS, Shi HL, Huang F, *et al.* (2016) Astragaloside IV inhibits microglia activation via glucocorticoid receptor mediated signaling pathway. *Sci Rep* **6**: 19137.

39. Ren XS, Leng XY, Yang YG, Xu XX. (2006) Neuroprotective effect of astragalus root on experimental injury of spinal cord in rats. *Chinese Journal of Clinical Rehabilitation* **10**(7): 31–33.

40. Zhang J, Ma T. (2014) Neuroprotective function of astragalus injection on treatment of rats with acute spinal cord injury. *Journal of Clinical Medicine in Practice* **18**(24): 7–10.

41. Gu DM, Lu PH, Zhang K, *et al.* (2015) EGFR mediates astragaloside IV-induced Nrf2 activation to protect cortical neurons against in vitro ischemia/reperfusion damages. *Biochem Biophys Res Commun* **457**(3): 391–397.

42. Xue B, Huang J, Ma B, *et al.* (2019) Astragaloside IV protects primary cerebral cortical neurons from oxygen and glucose deprivation/reoxygenation by activating the PKA/CREB pathway. *Neuroscience* **404**: 326–337.

43. Liu X, Zhang J, Wang S, *et al.* (2017) Astragaloside IV attenuates the H_2O_2-induced apoptosis of neuronal cells by inhibiting α-synuclein expression via the p38 MAPK pathway. *Int J Mol Med* **40**(6): 1772–1780.

44. Yue R, Li X, Chen B, *et al.* (2015) Astragaloside IV attenuates glutamate-induced neurotoxicity in PC12 cells through Raf-MEK-ERK pathway. *PLoS One* **10**(5): e0126603.

45. Guo C, Tong L, Xi M, *et al.* (2012) Neuroprotective effect of calycosin on cerebral ischemia and reperfusion injury in rats. *J Ethnopharmacol* **144**(3): 768–774.

46. Guo C, Ma Y, Ma S, *et al.* (2017) The role of TRPC6 in the neuroprotection of calycosin against cerebral ischemic injury. *Sci Rep* **7**(1): 3039.

47. Zhang H, Pan N, Xiong S, *et al.* (2012) Inhibition of polyglutamine-mediated proteotoxicity by Astragalus membranaceus polysaccharide through the DAF-16/FOXO transcription factor in Caenorhabditis elegans. *Biochem J* **441**(1): 417–424.

48. Maresca M, Micheli L, Cinci L, *et al.* (2017) Pain relieving and protective effects of Astragalus hydroalcoholic extract in rat arthritis models. *J Pharm Pharmacol* **69**(12): 1858–1870.

49. Wu XL, Wang YY, Cheng J, Zhao YY. (2006) Calcium channel blocking activity of calycosin, a major active component of Astragali Radix, on rat aorta. *Acta Pharmacol Sin* **27**(8): 1007–1012.

50. Revuelta MP, Cantabrana B, Hidalgo A. (2000) Mechanisms involved in kaempferol-induced relaxation in rat uterine smooth muscle. *Life Sci* **67**(3): 251–259.

51. Zhang C, Fan L, Fan S, *et al.* (2019) Cinnamomum cassia presl: A review of its traditional uses, phytochemistry, pharmacology and toxicology. *Molecules* **24**(19) pii: E3473.

52. Ho SC, Chang KS, Chang PW. (2013) Inhibition of neuroinflammation by cinnamon and its main components. *Food Chem* **138**(4): 2275–2282.

53. Fu Y, Yang P, Zhao Y, *et al.* (2017) Trans-cinnamaldehyde inhibits microglial activation and improves neuronal survival against neuroinflammation in BV2 microglial cells with lipopolysaccharide stimulation. *Evid Based Complement Alternat Med* **2017**: 4730878.

54. Zhang L, Zhang Z, Fu Y, *et al.* (2016) Trans-cinnamaldehyde improves memory impairment by blocking microglial activation through the destabilization of iNOS mRNA in mice challenged with lipopolysaccharide. *Neuropharmacology* **110**(Pt A): 503–518.

55. Zhao Y, Deng H, Li K, *et al.* (2019) Trans-cinnamaldehyde improves neuroinflammation-mediated NMDA receptor dysfunction and memory deficits through blocking NF-κB pathway in presenilin1/2 conditional double knockout mice. *Brain Behav Immun* **82**: 45–62.

56. Hwang H, Jeon H, Ock J, *et al.* (2011) 2'-Hydroxycinnamaldehyde targets low-density lipoprotein receptor-related protein-1 to inhibit lipopolysaccharide-induced microglial activation. *J Neuroimmunol* **230**(1–2): 52–64.

57. Frydman-Marom A, Levin A, Farfara D, *et al.* (2011) Orally administrated cinnamon extract reduces β-amyloid oligomerization and corrects cognitive impairment in Alzheimer's disease animal models. *PLoS One* **6**(1): e16564.

58. Zeng GJ, Huang HC, Li Y. (2017) Protective effect of total flavonoids of cinnamomi cortex on PC12 cell injured by 6-hydroxydopamine. *J Chin Med Mater* **40**: 2936–2940.

59. Kim C, Lee JH, Kim W, *et al.* (2016) The suppressive effects of cinnamomi cortex and its phytocompound coumarin on oxaliplatin-induced neuropathic cold allodynia in rats. *Molecules* **21**(9): 1253.

60. Chae HK, Kim W, Kim SK. (2019) Phytochemicals of cinnamomi cortex: Cinnamic acid, but not cinnamaldehyde, attenuates oxaliplatin-induced cold and mechanical hypersensitivity in rats. *Nutrients* **11**(2): 432.

61. Sun L, Zong SB, Li JC, *et al.* (2016) The essential oil from the twigs of Cinnamomum cassia Presl alleviates pain and inflammation in mice. *J Ethnopharmacol* **194**: 904–912.

62. Chen Z, Zhang C, Gao F, *et al.* (2018) A systematic review on the rhizome of ligusticum chuanxiong Hort. (*chuanxiong*). *Food Chem Toxicol* **119**: 309–325.

63. Or TC, Yang CL, Law AH, *et al.* (2011) Isolation and identification of anti-inflammatory constituents from ligusticum *chuanxiong* and their underlying mechanisms of action on microglia. *Neuropharmacology* **60**(6): 823–831.

64. Luo Y, Li X, Liu T, *et al.* (2019) Senkyunolide H protects against MPP(+)-induced apoptosis via the ROS-mediated mitogen-activated

protein kinase pathway in PC12 cells. *Environ Toxicol Pharmacol* **65**: 73–81.

65. Kim M, Kim SO, Lee M, *et al.* (2014) Tetramethylpyrazine, a natural alkaloid, attenuates pro-inflammatory mediators induced by amyloid beta and interferon-gamma in rat brain microglia. *Eur J Pharmacol* **740**: 504–511.

66. Cheng CY, Ho TY, Lee EJ, *et al.* (2008) Ferulic acid reduces cerebral infarct through its antioxidative and anti-inflammatory effects following transient focal cerebral ischemia in rats. *Am J Chin Med* **36**(6): 1105–1119.

67. Nam KN, Kim KP, Cho KH, *et al.* (2013) Prevention of inflammation-mediated neurotoxicity by butylidenephthalide and its role in microglial activation. *Cell Biochem Funct* **31**(8): 707–712.

68. Wu XM, Qian ZM, Zhu L, *et al.* (2011) Neuroprotective effect of ligustilide against ischaemia–reperfusion injury via up-regulation of erythropoietin and down-regulation of RTP801. *Br J Pharmacol* **164**(2): 332–343.

69. Chen Z, Pan X, Georgakilas AG, *et al.* (2013) Tetramethylpyrazine (TMP) protects cerebral neurocytes and inhibits glioma by down regulating chemokine receptor CXCR4 expression. *Cancer Lett* **336**(2): 281–289.

70. Li SY, Jia YH, Sun WG, *et al.* (2010) Stabilization of mitochondrial function by tetramethylpyrazine protects against kainate-induced oxidative lesions in the rat hippocampus. *Free Radic Biol Med* **48**(4): 597–608.

71. Lu C, Zhang J, Shi X, *et al.* (2014) Neuroprotective effects of tetramethylpyrazine against dopaminergic neuron injury in a rat model of Parkinson's disease induced by MPTP. *Int J Biol Sci* **10**(4): 350–357.

72. Fan L, Wang K, Shi Z, *et al.* (2011) Tetramethylpyrazine protects spinal cord and reduces inflammation in a rat model of spinal cord ischemia–reperfusion injury. *J Vasc Surg* **54**(1): 192–200.

73. Bie BH, Chen Y, Zhao ZQ. (2006) Ligustrazine inhibits high voltage-gated Ca(2+) and TTX-resistant Na(+) channels of primary sensory neuron and thermal nociception in the rat: A study on peripheral mechanism. *Neurosci Bull* **22**(2): 79–84.

74. Jiang L, Pan CL, Wang CY, *et al.* (2017) Selective suppression of the JNK-MMP2/9 signal pathway by tetramethylpyrazine attenuates neuropathic pain in rats. *J Neuroinflammation* **14**(1): 174.

75. Peng C, Xie X, Wang L, *et al.* (2009) Pharmacodynamic action and mechanism of volatile oil from Rhizoma Ligustici Chuanxiong Hort. on treating headache. *Phytomedicine* **16**(1): 25–34.

76. Ozaki Y, Sekita S, Harada M. (1989) Centrally acting muscle relaxant effect of phthalides (ligustilide, cnidilide and senkyunolide) obtained from Cnidium officinale Makino (article in Japanese). *Yakugaku Zasshi* **109**(6): 402–406.

77. Xie XQ, Zhan K, Yin RL, Yang LH. (2007) Advances in studies on volatile oil of ligusticum chuanxiong Hort. *Lishizhen Med Mater Med Res* **18**: 1508–1510.

78. Wei WL, Zeng R, Gu CM, *et al.* (2016) Angelica sinensis in China — A review of botanical profile, ethnopharmacology, phytochemistry and chemical analysis. *J Ethnopharmacol* **190**: 116–141.

79. Xie Y, Zhang H, Zhang Y, *et al.* (2018) Chinese Angelica Polysaccharide (CAP) alleviates LPS-induced inflammation and apoptosis by down-regulating COX-1 in PC12 cells. *Cell Physiol Biochem* **49**(4): 1380–1388.

80. Yu Y, Du JR, Wang CY, Qian ZM. (2008) Protection against hydrogen peroxide-induced injury by Z-ligustilide in PC12 cells. *Exp Brain Res* **184**(3): 307–312.

81. Kuang X, Yao Y, Du JR, *et al.* (2006) Neuroprotective role of Z-ligustilide against forebrain ischemic injury in ICR mice. *Brain Res* **1102**(1): 145–153.

82. Kuang X, Wang LF, Yu L, *et al.* (2014) Ligustilide ameliorates neuroinflammation and brain injury in focal cerebral ischemia/reperfusion rats: Involvement of inhibition of TLR4/peroxiredoxin 6 signaling. *Free Radic Biol Med* **71**: 165–175.

83. Song M, Li QX, He C. (2009) Identification and analgesic effect of Angelica sinensis extract. *Journal of Xianning University* **23**: 194–196.

84. Zhang A, Xu C, Liang S, *et al.* (2008) Role of sodium ferulate in the nociceptive sensory facilitation of neuropathic pain injury mediated by P2X(3) receptor. *Neurochem Int* **53**(6–8): 278–282.

85. Xu Y, Zhang L, Shao T, *et al.* (2013) Ferulic acid increases pain threshold and ameliorates depression-like behaviors in reserpine-treated mice: Behavioral and neurobiological analyses. *Metab Brain Dis* **28**(4): 571–583.

86. Xu Y, Lin D, Yu X, *et al.* (2016) The antinociceptive effects of ferulic acid on neuropathic pain: Involvement of descending monoaminergic system and opioid receptors. *Oncotarget* **7**(15): 20455–20468.

87. Ko WC. (1980) A newly isolated antispasmodic — butylidenephthalide. *Jpn J Pharmacol* **30**(1): 85–91.

88. Asl MN, Hosseinzadeh H. (2008) Review of pharmacological effects of Glycyrrhiza sp. and its bioactive compounds. *Phytother Res* **22**(6): 709–724.

89. Park SH, Kang JS, Yoon YD, *et al.* (2010) Glabridin inhibits lipopolysaccharide-induced activation of a microglial cell line, BV-2, by blocking NF-κB and AP-1. *Phytother Res* **24**(Suppl 1): S29–S34.

90. Song JH, Lee JW, Shim B, *et al.* (2013) Glycyrrhizin alleviates neuroinflammation and memory deficit induced by systemic lipopolysaccharide treatment in mice. *Molecules* **18**(12): 15788–15803.

91. Yu JY, Ha JY, Kim KM, *et al.* (2015) Anti-inflammatory activities of licorice extract and its active compounds, glycyrrhizic acid, liquiritin and liquiritigenin, in BV2 cells and mice liver. *Molecules* **20**(7): 13041–13054.

92. Liu W, Huang S, Li Y, *et al.* (2019) Suppressive effect of glycyrrhizic acid against lipopolysaccharide-induced neuroinflammation and cognitive impairment in C57 mice via toll-like receptor 4 signaling pathway. *Food Nutr Res* **63**: 1516.

93. Yang EJ, Min JS, Ku HY, *et al.* (2012) Isoliquiritigenin isolated from Glycyrrhiza uralensis protects neuronal cells against glutamate-induced mitochondrial dysfunction. *Biochem Biophys Res Commun* **421**(4): 658–664.

94. Lee HK, Yang EJ, Kim JY, *et al.* (2012) Inhibitory effects of Glycyrrhizae radix and its active component, isoliquiritigenin, on $A\beta$(25–35)-induced neurotoxicity in cultured rat cortical neurons. *Arch Pharm Res* **35**(5): 897–904.

95. Zhan C, Yang J. (2006) Protective effects of isoliquiritigenin in transient middle cerebral artery occlusion-induced focal cerebral ischemia in rats. *Pharmacol Res* **53**(3): 303–309.

96. Sun YX, Tang Y, Wu AL, *et al.* (2010) Neuroprotective effect of liquiritin against focal cerebral ischemia/reperfusion in mice via its antioxidant and antiapoptosis properties. *J Asian Nat Prod Res* **12**(12): 1051–1060.

97. Shi Y, Wu D, Sun Z, *et al.* (2012) Analgesic and uterine relaxant effects of isoliquiritigenin, a flavone from Glycyrrhiza glabra. *Phytother Res* **26**(9): 1410–1417.

98. Zhang MT, Wang B, Jia YN, *et al.* (2017) Neuroprotective effect of liquiritin against neuropathic pain induced by chronic constriction injury of the sciatic nerve in mice. *Biomed Pharmacother* **95**: 186–198.

99. Zhang LL, Tian K, Tang ZH, *et al.* (2016) Phytochemistry and pharmacology of carthamus tinctorius L. *Am J Chin Med* **44**(2): 197–226.

100. Zhang Z, Wu Z, Zhu X, *et al.* (2014) Hydroxy-safflor yellow A inhibits neuroinflammation mediated by $A\beta_{1-42}$ in BV-2 cells. *Neurosci Lett* **562**: 39–44.

101. Lv Y, Qian Y, Ou-Yang A, Fu L. (2016) Hydroxysafflor yellow A attenuates neuron damage by suppressing the lipopolysaccharide-induced TLR4 pathway in activated microglial cells. *Cell Mol Neurobiol* **36**(8): 1241–1256.

102. Wang T, Ding YX, He J, *et al.* (2018) Hydroxysafflor yellow A attenuates lipopolysaccharide-induced neurotoxicity and neuroinflammation in primary mesencephalic cultures. *Molecules* **23**(5): 1210.

103. Han B, Zhao H. (2010) Effects of hydroxysafflor yellow A in the attenuation of MPTP neurotoxicity in mice. *Neurochem Res* **35**(1): 107–113.

104. Yang Q, Yang ZF, Liu SB, *et al.* (2010) Neuroprotective effects of hydroxysafflor yellow A against excitotoxic neuronal death partially through down-regulation of NR2B-containing NMDA receptors. *Neurochem Res* **35**(9): 1353–1360.

105. Kong SZ, Xian YF, Ip SP, *et al.* (2013) Protective effects of hydroxysafflor yellow A on beta-amyloid-induced neurotoxicity in PC12 cells. *Neurochem Res* **38**(5): 951–960.

106. Fu PK, Pan TL, Yang CY, *et al.* (2016) Carthamus tinctorius L. ameliorates brain injury followed by cerebral ischemia–reperfusion in rats by antioxidative and anti-inflammatory mechanisms. *Iran J Basic Med Sci* **19**(12): 1368–1375.

107. Shan LQ, Ma S, Qiu XC, *et al.* (2010) Hydroxysafflor yellow A protects spinal cords from ischemia/reperfusion injury in rabbits. *BMC Neurosci* **11**: 98.

108. Yu L, Chen C, Wang LF, *et al.* (2013) Neuroprotective effect of kaempferol glycosides against brain injury and neuroinflammation by inhibiting the activation of NF-κB and STAT3 in transient focal stroke. *PLoS One* **8**(2): e55839.

109. Popov AM, Li IA, Kang DI. (2009) Analgesic properties of CF extracted from the safflor (carthamus tinctorius) seeds and its potential uses. *Pharm Chem J* **43**(1): 41–44.

110. Wang Y, Chen P, Tang C, *et al.* (2014) Antinociceptive and anti-inflammatory activities of extract and two isolated flavonoids of Carthamus tinctorius L. *J Ethnopharmacol* **151**(2): 944–950.

111. Azietaku JT, Ma H, Yu XA, *et al.* (2017) A review of the ethnopharmacology, phytochemistry and pharmacology of Notopterygium incisum. *J Ethnopharmacol* **202**: 241–255.

112. Zschocke S, Lehner M, Bauer R. (1997) 5-Lipoxygenase and cyclooxygenase inhibitory active constituents from *Qianghuo* (Notopterygium incisum). *Planta Med* **63**(3): 203–206.

113. Okuyama E, Nishimura S, Ohmori S, *et al.* (1993) Analgesic component of Notopterygium incisum Ting. *Chem Pharm Bull (Tokyo)* **41**(5): 926–929.

114. Tang RN, Qu XB, Guan SH, *et al.* (2012) Chemical constituents of Spatholobus suberectus. *Chin J Nat Med* **10**(1): 32–35.

115. Zhang R, Liu C, Liu X, Guo Y. (2016) Protective effect of Spatholobus suberectus on brain tissues in cerebral ischemia. *Am J Transl Res* **8**(9): 3963–3969.

116. Park HR, Lee H, Lee JJ, *et al.* (2018) Protective effects of Spatholobi Caulis extract on neuronal damage and focal ischemic stroke/reperfusion injury. *Mol Neurobiol* **55**(6): 4650–4666.

117. Tian Z, Liu SB, Wang YC, *et al.* (2013) Neuroprotective effects of formononetin against NMDA-induced apoptosis in cortical neurons. *Phytother Res* **27**(12): 1770–1775.

7

Clinical Evidence for Acupuncture Therapies

OVERVIEW

This chapter provides a synopsis of the clinical evidence of acupuncture therapies used to manage cervical radiculopathy. A number of acupuncture therapies have been evaluated by clinical studies, including body acupuncture, electroacupuncture, moxibustion, warm needling, abdominal acupuncture and ear acupuncture. Evidence from these clinical studies has been summarised. Frequently used acupuncture points are listed.

Introduction

This chapter evaluates the clinical evidence on acupuncture therapies for cervical radiculopathy (CR). Acupuncture therapies refer to a group of therapies that stimulate certain acupuncture points, including body acupuncture (commonly called acupuncture), electroacupuncture, moxibustion and some special types of acupuncture. Following consistent methods of database searching and study screening as in the Chinese herbal medicine (CHM) studies (see Chapter 5), systematic reviews and clinical trials of acupuncture-related therapies for CR are summarised and synthesised in this chapter.

Previous Systematic Reviews

Three systematic reviews were identified from our comprehensive search.[1-3] All of these three systematic reviews evaluated the effects of acupuncture using traction therapy as the comparator, as well as the add-on effects of acupuncture to traction therapy, a commonly used physiotherapy method in clinical practice.

Sun *et al.*'s study in 2009 systematically reviewed randomised controlled trials (RCTs) of acupuncture therapies using traction therapy as the comparator.[1] Eight RCTs were included in this review, with five studies comparing acupuncture therapies with traction therapy and the other three RCTs evaluating the add-on effects of acupuncture to a combination of traction and *tuina* 推拿 therapies. Acupuncture therapies included body acupuncture, electroacupuncture and abdominal acupuncture. Meta-analysis results from four RCTs showed that acupuncture therapies were more effective than traction therapy in terms of total effective rate; however, the authors did not separate studies according to different acupuncture methods. In terms of the outcome measures of pain, meta-analysis of two RCTs showed that acupuncture therapies were more effective than traction therapy for the pain Visual Analogue Scale (VAS), but there was no difference between acupuncture therapies and traction therapy for the Pain Rating Index (PRI) of the McGill Pain Questionnaire (MPQ). The authors did not draw a firm conclusion due to the small number of studies for each comparison and their weakness in methodological quality.

A total of 14 RCTs were included in Hu *et al.*'s study in 2012.[2] Six studies compared acupuncture or electroacupuncture with traction therapy and the other eight studies evaluated the add-on effects of acupuncture or electroacupuncture to traction therapy. The Cochrane risk-of-bias assessment approach was used to assess the methodological quality of the included RCTs. Meta-analyses were conducted on the outcome measure of the total effective rate according to the different comparisons. It was found that acupuncture was more effective than traction therapy and adding acupuncture to traction therapy was more effective than traction therapy alone. However, the low methodological quality was the main concern with all included studies and prevented the authors from making a conclusion.

Yin *et al.*'s study in 2018 systematically reviewed the efficacy and safety of acupuncture for CR using traction therapy as the comparator.[3] Eleven RCTs were included in this review, including eight studies comparing acupuncture with traction therapy and three studies evaluating the add-on effects of acupuncture to traction therapy. The Cochrane risk-of-bias assessment and Jadad scale were used to assess the methodological quality of the included RCTs. Meta-analyses on the outcome measures of the pain VAS and MPQ scores showed favourable effects of acupuncture. However, the authors did not separate the different comparisons in the meta-analyses. The authors also pointed out that the low methodological quality of the included RCTs was of concern.

Identification of Clinical Studies

A comprehensive search of nine databases identified 20,537 citations, of which 4,369 required full-text retrieval to determine their eligibility for inclusion (Fig. 7.1). After assessment against rigorous inclusion criteria, 48 articles relating to 46 clinical studies that evaluated acupuncture-related therapies for CR were included.

A total of 25 articles (A1–A25) reporting the results of 23 RCTs met our inclusion criteria. Three articles (A5–A7) reported different outcomes of the same study; these were merged into one study in our analysis. Twenty-four articles were published in Chinese and one in English. Furthermore, 21 non-controlled studies were also included in our evaluation (A26–A46).

Among all studies, the acupuncture therapies included body acupuncture, electroacupuncture, moxibustion, warm needling (a combination of acupuncture needling and moxibustion), auricular acupuncture, abdominal examination, dermal acupuncture, and other special types of acupuncture.

In addition, 16 studies evaluated acupuncture-type therapies that are not commonly practised outside China; these studies are not introduced in this chapter.

Randomised Controlled Trials

In total, 25 articles (A1 to A25) reporting on 23 RCTs were included according to the selection criteria (Fig. 7.1), with 24 articles published

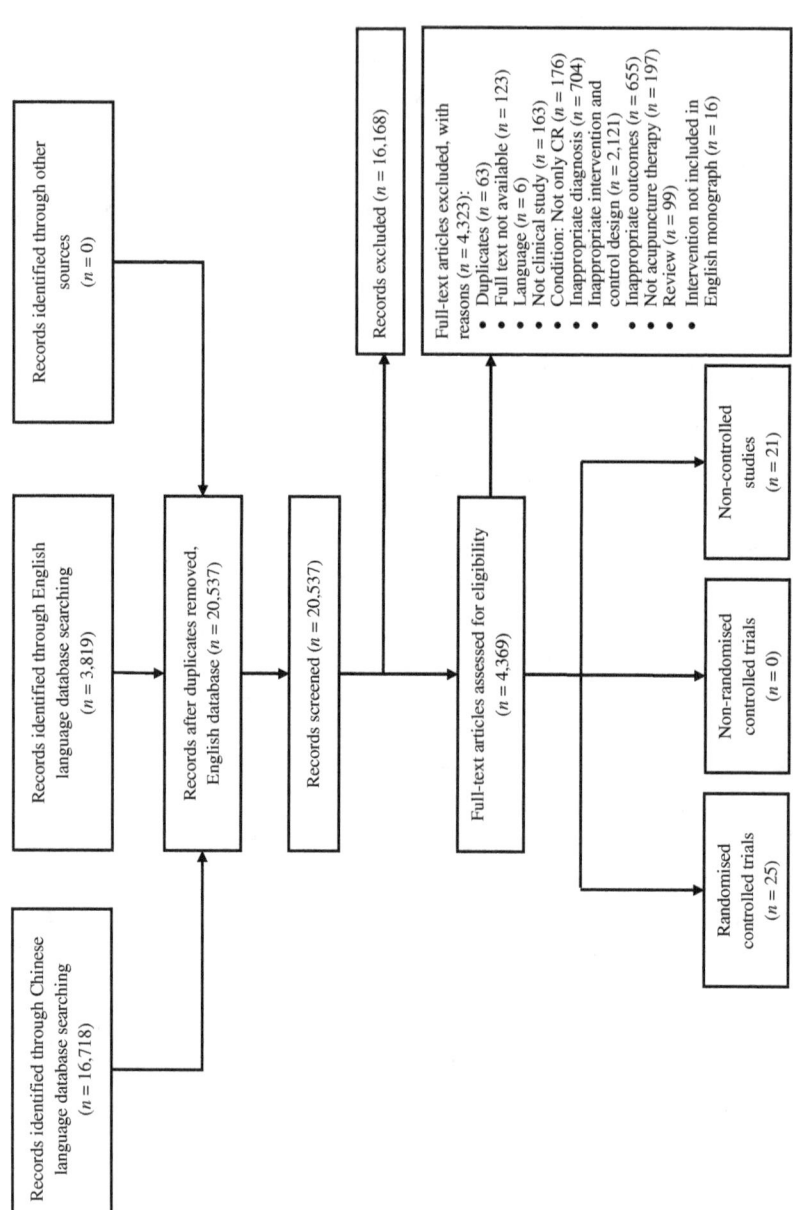

Fig. 7.1. Flow chart of the study selection process: Acupuncture-related therapies.

in Chinese and another one in the English language (A25). Three articles reported different outcomes of one RCT (A5–A7); the results of these three studies were merged in our analyses.

A total of 2,292 participants were included in the 23 studies. The age of participants ranged from 21 (A25) to 72 (A2) years, with a disease duration ranging from two days (A15) to 25 years (A3). Chinese medicine syndrome differentiation was mentioned in two studies (A4, A25), with the common syndromes being: Wind-cold-dampness 风寒湿, *qi* and Blood deficiency 气血亏虚, phlegm-dampness blocking meridians 痰湿阻络 and Liver-Kidney deficiency 肝肾不足. Both studies applied individually modified treatment methods according to Chinese medicine syndromes in addition to standardised basic treatments.

The most frequently used acupuncture points reported in these RCTs were: Cervical EX-B2 *Jiaji* points 颈夹脊穴 (*n* = 11), GV14 *Dazhui* 大椎 (*n* = 10), GB20 *Fengchi* 风池 (*n* = 7), CV12 *Zhongwan* 中脘 (*n* = 5), CV4 *Guanyuan* 关元 (*n* = 5), BL10 *Tianzhu* 天柱 (*n* = 5), *Ashi* points 阿是穴 (*n* = 5), SI3 *Houxi* 后溪 (*n* = 4), BL11 *Dazhu* 大杼 (*n* = 4) and EX-HN15 *Jing bailao* 颈百劳 (*n* = 4).

Among these 23 RCTs, one study (A25) compared body acupuncture with sham acupuncture, 16 (A2, A3, A5–A7, A9, A10, A12–A19, A21, A22, A24) studies compared certain types of acupuncture therapies with routine care therapies and the other six studies (A1, A4, A8, A11, A20, A23) compared a combination of acupuncture therapies plus routine care therapies with routine care therapies alone.

The types of acupuncture therapies evaluated were:

- Body acupuncture: Nine studies (A1, A3, A5–A7, A15, A17, A19, A22, A23, A25);
- Electroacupuncture: Five studies (A2, A9, A10, A14, A21);
- Moxibustion: One study (A4);
- Warm needling: One study (A20);
- Abdominal acupuncture 腹针: Four studies (A8, A11, A12, A18); and

- Other types of acupuncture:

  - "Stuck needle acupuncture" 滞动针 plus electroacupuncture: One study (A24);
  - Body acupuncture plus dermal acupuncture: One study (A13); and
  - Electroacupuncture plus auricular acupuncture: One study (A16).

It is worth mentioning that Wei's study (A4) in 2009 used moxibustion sticks on acupuncture points, which is a common moxibustion therapy, while Lin's study (A20) in 2017 applied moxibustion cones stuck on the handles of acupuncture needles, which is a combination of acupuncture and moxibustion. The latter is named "warm needling" in this study.

Abdominal acupuncture 腹针 therapy was investigated in four studies (A8, A11, A12, A18). Abdominal acupuncture was invented by Prof. Bo Zhi-yun in 1972 based on the theory of "wholistic" treatment. In this therapy, the abdominal area is considered a micro-system of the whole body and that stimulating certain points in the abdominal region will produce therapeutic effects for a number of clinical conditions.[4] Of these four RCTs, two studies (A12, A18) compared abdominal acupuncture with traction therapy and the other two studies (A8, A11) evaluated the add-on effects of abdominal acupuncture to traction therapy.

In addition, other types of unconventional acupuncture therapies were identified, such as "stuck needle" acupuncture 滞动针 (A24). When performing "stuck needle" acupuncture 滞动针, the practitioner will wind the needle towards one direction to make the needle stick, then pull or shake the needle to move the tissues around it.

One RCT compared acupuncture with sham acupuncture; 16 studies compared acupuncture therapies with routine care therapies, including pharmacotherapy, traction therapy, physiotherapy or their combinations; the other six studies evaluated the add-on effects of acupuncture therapies to routine care therapies.

Outcome measures reported by the included studies were: The effective rate ($n = 19$), pain VAS or NRS ($n = 13$), Short-Form Mcgill Pain Questionnaire (SF-MPQ) ($n = 6$), Northwick Park Neck Pain Questionnaire (NPR) ($n = 3$), Scoring System for Cervical Radiculopathy

(SSCR) (n = 3), Short Form (36) Health Survey (SF-36) (n = 3), Neck Disability Index (NDI) (n = 1) and Clinical Assessment Scale for Cervical Spondylosis (CASCS) (n = 1).

Risk-of-Bias Assessment of Included Randomised Controlled Trials

Among all the included studies (n = 23), 13 studies stated appropriate methods for sequence generation of random numbers and therefore were assessed as "low" risk of bias for this domain, while the other 11 studies were of "unclear" risk of bias due to a lack of information.

For allocation concealment, three studies were assessed as "low" risk of bias since they applied the opaque envelope method and the other studies were of "unclear" risk due to a lack of information.

One study applied sham acupuncture as the control method but did not mention any effort at blinding, so we assessed this study as an "unclear" risk for blinding of participants; the other studies were all of "high" risk of bias for this item. Considering that acupuncture is a physical intervention, the acupuncturist who delivers treatments must be aware of the allocation so all studies were judged as "high" risk for the blinding of personnel. In terms of the blinding of outcome assessors, only the sham control study was of "unclear" risk of bias because it is possible that participants reported all subjective outcomes, while the other studies were at "high" risk of bias since both participants and practitioners were aware of group allocation.

Incomplete outcome data was assessed as "low" risk of bias for all studies. All studies were assessed as "unclear" risk for selective reporting, as protocols could not be identified for any studies. See Table 7.1 for a summary.

Overall Treatment Effects of Acupuncture Therapies

When merging all different types of acupuncture therapies, meta-analyses results show that on the whole, acupuncture therapy was more effective than overall routine care therapies or traction therapy only, in terms of the outcome measures of the effective rate, pain VAS, MPQ total score, MPQ Pain Rating Index (PRI) score, and MPQ

Table 7.1.   Risk-of-Bias Assessment of Randomised Controlled Trials

Risk-of-Bias Domain	Low Risk *n* (%)	Unclear Risk *n* (%)	High Risk *n* (%)
Sequence generation	13 (56.5)	10 (43.5)	0 (0)
Allocation concealment	3 (13)	20 (87)	0 (0)
Blinding of participants	0 (0)	1 (4.3)	22 (95.7)
Blinding of personnel*	0 (0)	0 (0)	23 (100)
Blinding of outcome assessors	0 (0)	1 (4.3)	22 (95.7)
Incomplete outcome data	23 (100)	0 (0)	0 (0)
Selective outcome reporting	0 (0)	23 (100)	0 (0)

*Blinding of personnel is challenging in manual therapies.

Present Pain Intensity (PPI) score. In addition, the meta-analysis also showed that acupuncture was an effective add-on therapy to overall routine care therapies or traction therapy for the outcome measures of the effective rate and pain VAS. Results are shown in Table 7.2.

Considering that the acupuncture therapies used in the included studies varied greatly, it is critical to analyse the studies according to the different acupuncture therapies. Therefore, the treatment effects of each therapy are presented separately in line with the comparisons and outcome measures, as follows.

Body Acupuncture

Body Acupuncture vs. Sham Acupuncture

One RCT (A25) compared body acupuncture with sham acupuncture, with infrared radiation used in both groups as the co-intervention. A total of 117 participants enrolled in this RCT (59 received real acupuncture *vs.* 58 receiving sham acupuncture). The treatment effects were evaluated using the pain VAS and the NPQ. Results showed that real acupuncture was significantly more effective than sham acupuncture for both outcome measures, at both the end of treatment and the follow-up phases.

Table 7.2. Meta-Analyses Results for Combined Acupuncture Therapies

Outcome	Comparison	No. of Studies (Participants)	Effect Size (RR or MD: [95% CI], I²)	Included Studies
Effective rate	Overall: Acupuncture *vs.* routine care therapies	12 (1,437)	RR: 1.16 [1.11, 1.21]*, 6%	A3, A5, A10, A12, A14, A15, A17–A19, A21, A22, A24
	Subgroup: Acupuncture *vs.* traction therapy	8 (814)	RR: 1.19 [1.13, 1.25]*, 0%	A3, A5, A10, A12, A15, A18, A19, A21
	Acupuncture *vs.* pharmacotherapy	3 (533)	RR: 1.10 [1.04, 1.16]*, 0%	A22, A14, A24
	Overall: Acupuncture add-on to routine care therapies	6 (479)	RR: 1.14 [1.03, 1.27]*, 64%	A1, A4, A8, A11, A20, A23
	Subgroup: Acupuncture add-on to traction therapy	5 (389)	RR: 1.17 [1.02, 1.35]*, 73%	A1, A4, A8, A11, A20
VAS/NRS	Overall: Acupuncture *vs.* routine care therapies	8 (539)	MD: −1.26 [−1.79, −0.74]*, 88%	A22, A24, A6, A10, A15, A19, A17, A9
	Subgroup: Acupuncture *vs.* traction therapy	5 (364)	MD: −1.24 [−1.54, −0.93]*, 27%	A6, A10, A13, A15, A19
	Overall: Acupuncture add-on to routine care therapies	4 (308)	MD: −1.25 [−1.66, −0.84]*, 79%	A1, A8, A20, A23
	Subgroup: Acupuncture add-on to traction therapy	3 (218)	MD: −1.07 [−1.35, −0.79]*, 51%	A1, A8, A20
MPQ total score	Acupuncture *vs.* traction therapy	2 (129))	MD: −3.67 [−5.66, −1.69]*, 81%	A13, A16
MPQ PRI	Overall: Acupuncture *vs.* routine care therapies	5 (362)	MD: −2.24 [−3.64, −0.85]*, 89%	A6, A10, A13, A15, A22
	Subgroup: Acupuncture *vs.* traction therapy	4 (304)	MD: −2.08 [−3.57, −0.60]*, 92%	A6, A10, A13, A15

(Continued)

Table 7.2. (*Continued*)

Outcome	Comparison	No. of Studies (Participants)	Effect Size (RR or MD: [95% CI], I²)	Included Studies
MPQ PPI	Overall: Acupuncture *vs.* routine care therapies	5 (362)	MD: −0.46 [−0.64, −0.28]*, 36%	A6, A10, A13, A15, A22
	Subgroup: Acupuncture *vs.* traction therapy	4 (304)	MD: −0.42 [−0.62, −0.22]*, 40%	A6, A10, A13, A15

Abbreviations: CI, confidence interval; MD, mean difference; MPQ, McGill Pain Questionnaire; NRS, Numeric Rating Scale; PPI, Present Pain Intensity; PRI, Pain Rating Index; RR, risk ratio; VAS, Visual Analogue Scale.
*Statistically significant.

Body Acupuncture vs. Routine Care Therapies

Six studies (A3, A5–A7, A15, A17, A19, A22) evaluated the treatment effects of body acupuncture with different routine care therapies as comparators. A total of 480 participants were included in these studies.

Among the six studies, one study (A22) compared acupuncture on cervical EX-B2 *Jiaji* points 颈夹脊穴 with pharmacotherapy (indomethacin and vit B) on 60 participants. The treatment duration was 10 days. The outcome measures used in this study were the effective rate, pain VAS, NDI, MPQ and SF-36.

Four RCTs compared acupuncture with traction therapy (A3, A5–A7, A15, A19). Of these, Wang's study (A5–A7) in 2014 applied an acupuncture technique named "neck eight needles" 项八针, referring to needling eight points in the cervical region: GV14 *Dazhui* 大椎, GV15 *Yamen* 哑门 and two *cun* 寸 besides the posterior midline at the C2, C4 and C6 levels bilaterally. The sixty participants involved in this study received acupuncture or traction therapy for two weeks. Outcomes reported by this study were the effective rate (A5), pain VAS and MPQ (A6) and SF-36 (A7). One study (A15) applied a point-to-point needling technique on four pairs of points on the affected side: Cervical EX-B2 *Jiaji* points 颈夹脊穴 from C4 to C7 levels, from SI14 *Jianwaishu* 肩外俞 to SI13 *Quyuan* 曲垣, from SI11 *Tianzong* 天宗 to SI10 *Naoshu* 臑俞 and from LI10 *Shousanli* 手三里 to LI8

Xialian 下廉. Both acupuncture and the traction therapy were applied once a day for two weeks. The effective rate, pain VAS and MPQ were used as outcome measures in this study. Another study compared acupuncture therapy with an electronic treatment instrument for a 10-day treatment, using the effective rate, pain VAS and SSCR as outcome measures.

In terms of the total effective rate, overall meta-analysis of these six studies showed that acupuncture therapies were superior to routine care therapies (6 studies, RR: 1.21 [1.13, 1.30], I^2 = 0%) (A3, A5, A15, A17, A19, A22). Subgroup analysis also showed that acupuncture therapies were more effective than traction therapy (4 studies, RR: 1.21 [1.12, 1.32], I^2 = 0%) (A3, A5, A15, A19). On the other hand, there was only a single study on acupuncture compared with pharmacotherapy or an electronic treatment instrument; the results could not be confirmed (see Table 7.3).

Table 7.3. **Acupuncture *vs.* Routine Care Therapies**

Outcome	Comparison	No. of Studies (Participants)	Effect Size (RR or MD: [95% CI], I^2)	Included Studies
Effective rate	Overall: Acupuncture *vs.* routine care therapies	6 (478)	RR: 1.21 [1.13, 1.30]*, 0%	A3, A5, A15, A17, A19, A22
	Subgroup: Acupuncture *vs.* traction therapy	4 (330)	RR: 1.21 [1.12, 1.32]*, 0%	A3, A5, A15, A19
VAS/NRS	Overall: Acupuncture *vs.* routine care therapies	5 (388)	MD: −1.57 [−2.04, −1.09]*, 78%	A6, A15, A7, A19, A22
	Subgroup: Acupuncture *vs.* traction therapy	3 (240)	MD: −1.33 [−1.71, −0.95]*, 35%	A6, A15, A19
MPQ PRI	Acupuncture *vs.* traction therapy	2 (180)	MD: −2.46 [−4.72, −0.19]*, 92%	A6, A15
MPQ PPI	Acupuncture *vs.* traction therapy	2 (180)	MD: −0.35 [−0.69, 0.00], 73%	A6, A15

(*Continued*)

Table 7.3. (*Continued*)

Outcome	Comparison	No. of Studies (Participants)	Effect Size (RR or MD: [95% CI], I²)	Included Studies
SF-36: Vitality	Overall: Acupuncture *vs.* routine care therapies	2 (120)	MD: −1.57 [−19.83, 16.69], 92%	A7, A22
SF-36: Physical functioning	Overall: Acupuncture *vs.* routine care therapies	2 (120)	MD: −3.83 [−9.62, 1.97], 35%	A7, A22
SF-36: Bodily pain	Overall: Acupuncture *vs.* routine care therapies	2 (120)	MD: 4.17 [−4.97, 13.31], 62%	A7, A22
SF-36: General health perceptions	Overall: Acupuncture *vs.* routine care therapies	2 (120)	MD: −5.34 [−18.68, 7.99], 82%	A7, A22
SF-36: Physical role functioning	Overall: Acupuncture *vs.* routine care therapies	2 (120)	MD: 6.42 [−0.32, 13.17], 82%	A7, A22
SF-36: Emotional role functioning	Overall: Acupuncture *vs.* routine care therapies	2 (120)	MD: −0.08 [−26.69, 26.52], 93%	A7, A22
SF-36: Social role functioning	Overall: Acupuncture *vs.* routine care therapies	2 (120)	MD: −0.91 [−19.94, 18.12], 90%	A7, A22
SF-36: Mental health	Overall: Acupuncture *vs.* routine care therapies	2 (120)	MD: −3.30 [−18.80, 12.20], 86%	A7, A22

Abbreviations: CI, confidence interval; MD, mean difference; MPQ, McGill Pain Questionnaire; NRS, Numeric Rating Scale; PPI, Present Pain Intensity; PRI, Pain Rating Index; RR, risk ratio; SF-36, Short Form (36) Health Survey; SSCR, Scoring System for Cervical Radiculopathy; VAS, Visual Analogue Scale.
*Statistically significant.

For pain VAS or NRS scores, overall meta-analysis showed that acupuncture therapies were more effective than routine care therapies (5 studies, MD: −1.57 [−2.04, −1.09], I² = 78%) (A6, A15, A7, A19, A22). Specifically, acupuncture was more effective than traction therapy in terms of pain score (3 studies, MD: −1.33 [−1.71, −0.95], $I^2 = 35\%$) (A6, A15, A19) (see Table 7.3). The effects of acupuncture compared with pharmacotherapy or an electronic treatment instrument were only shown by a single study.

- Acupuncture *vs.* pharmacotherapy: One study (A22);
- Acupuncture *vs.* traction therapy: Four studies (A3, A5–A7, A15, A19); and
- Acupuncture *vs.* physiotherapy: One study (A17).

Three studies (A6, A15, A22) reported data on the SF-MPQ. The overall meta-analysis shows that acupuncture was more effective than routine care for the PRI score (3 studies, MD: −2.69 [−4.60, −0.78], $I^2 = 84\%$) and PPI score (3 studies, MD: −0.43 [−0.71, −0.16], $I^2 = 62\%$). Subgroup analysis shows that when comparing acupuncture with traction therapy (A6, A15), acupuncture was more effective than traction therapy for the PRI score (2 studies, MD: −2.46 [−4.72, −0.19], $I^2 = 92\%$); however, the superior effect was not found in the PPI score (see Table 7.3).

Two studies (A7, A22) reported data on the SF-36. Meta-analyses showed that there was no significant difference between the acupuncture therapies and routine care therapies for all eight sections (see Table 7.3).

One study (A5) reported data on the NPQ, showing that body acupuncture was more effective than traction therapy.

Body Acupuncture Plus Routine Care Therapies vs. Routine Care Therapies

- Acupuncture add-on *vs.* traction therapy: One study (A1); and
- Acupuncture add-on *vs.* pharmacotherapy and traction therapy: One study (A23).

Two studies evaluated the add-on effects of acupuncture to routine care therapies. One RCT (A1) compared the combination of acupuncture and traction therapy with traction therapy alone. Ninety participants were included in this study and completed 10-day treatments of acupuncture plus traction therapy or traction therapy alone. Acupuncture was applied on only one point bilaterally — SI3 *Houxi* 后溪. This study reported data on the effective rate and pain VAS. Another study (A23) evaluated the add-on effects of acupuncture to the combination of diclofenac sodium sustained-release tablets and traction therapy on 90 participants; the treatment duration was 14 days. This study also reported data on the effective rate and pain VAS. Meta-analyses of these two studies showed that adding acupuncture to routine care therapies increased the effective rate (2 studies, RR: 1.11 [1.01, 1.23], I^2 = 0%) and pain VAS (2 studies, MD: −1.63 [−2.46, −0.80], I^2 = 88%).

Electroacupuncture

Five studies (A2, A9, A10, A14, A21) evaluated the treatment effects of electroacupuncture. Electroacupuncture was applied once daily, with a treatment duration ranging from 10 to 20 days. All five studies selected cervical EX-B2 *Jiaji* points 颈夹脊穴 for electroacupuncture, in combination with other points located on relevant meridians. The comparators of these five studies varied, with two studies (A10, A21) comparing electroacupuncture with traction therapy, one study (A2) comparing electroacupuncture with pharmacotherapy (meloxicam), one study (A9) comparing electroacupuncture with physiotherapy, and one study (A9) comparing electroacupuncture with the combination of traction therapy and physiotherapy. The outcome measures used in these five studies varied, with the effective rate and pain VAS being reported by multiple studies. Overall meta-analyses showed that electroacupuncture was more effective than routine care therapies for the effective rate (3 studies, RR: 1.14 [1.01, 1.27], I^2 = 44%) but not for the pain VAS (2 studies, MD: −0.59 [−2.23, 1.05], I^2 = 76%). Superior effects of electroacupuncture were also shown in single studies when comparing electroacupuncture with physiotherapy for the CASCS score (A2), MPQ PRI score and PPI score (A10), and for SSCR scores when comparing electroacupuncture with traction therapy (A21).

In addition, one study (A14) incorporated a follow-up phase of six months. At the end of the follow-up phase, the effective rate of the electroacupuncture group was significantly higher than that of the medication group (meloxicam), showing that electroacupuncture achieved long-term effects.

Moxibustion

One study (A4) evaluated the add-on effects of moxibustion to traction therapy. In this study, moxibustion was applied on GV14 *Dazhui*, GB20 *Fengchi* 风池 and ST36 *Zusanli* 足三里 for 20 days. In addition, all participants received traction therapy and were guided to apply different diet therapies and massage according to their Chinese medicine syndrome differentiation. This study reported data on the effective rate and SF-36; the latter showing that adding moxibustion was beneficial for patients' quality of life.

Warm Needling

One study (A20) evaluated the add-on effect of warm needling therapy to traction therapy. Warm needling therapy involves placing moxibustion cones on the handles of acupuncture needles during acupuncture therapy and can be interpreted as a combination of acupuncture and moxibustion. A total of 70 participants were included in this study; all of them received traction therapy three times a week for four weeks. The participants in the warm needling group received warm needling in addition to each traction therapy treatment. Data on the effective rate and pain NRS were reported at the end of the 12-week treatment phase and at the end of the three-month follow-up phase, showing that adding warm needling therapy to traction therapy was more effective than traction therapy alone at both time points.

Abdominal Acupuncture

Four studies evaluated abdominal acupuncture; two of them (A12, A18) compared abdominal acupuncture with traction therapy and the other two studies (A8, A11) compared a combination of abdominal acupuncture and traction therapy with traction therapy alone. The abdominal acupuncture was applied once a day for 10 or 20 days. The points used in these four studies were all located in the abdominal region: CV12 *Zhongwan* 中脘 (*n* = 4), CV4 *Guanyuan* 关元 (*n* = 4), KI18 *Shiguan* 石关 (*n* = 3), KI17 *Shangqu* 商曲 (*n* = 3), ST24 *Huaroumen* 滑肉门 (*n* = 3) and CV10 *Xiawan* 下脘 (*n* = 1).

Two studies (A12, A18) involving 380 participants compared abdominal acupuncture with traction therapy; both studies reported data on the effective rate as the outcome measure. Meta-analysis results showed that abdominal acupuncture was superior to traction therapy in terms of the effective rate (2 studies, RR: 1.17 [1.08, 1.26], I^2 = 8%).

Bo's study (A12) in 2005 also reported data on the effective rate at the end of the three-month follow-up phase, showing that the abdominal acupuncture was more effective than traction therapy three months after the treatment ceased.

Another two studies involving 151 participants evaluated the add-on effects of abdominal acupuncture to traction therapy. One study (A8) reported data on the effective rate and pain VAS and the other study (A11) reported the effective rate. Meta-analysis results showed that the add-on benefit in terms of the effective rate was not statistically significant (2 studies, RR: 1.16 [0.88, 1.53], I^2 = 77%).

"Stuck Needle" Acupuncture

One study included a special technique — "stuck needle" acupuncture (A24). Acupuncture was applied on cervical EX-B2 *Jiaji* points 颈夹脊穴, GB20 Fengchi 风池 and *Ashi* points 阿是穴. The "stuck needle" technique was performed to enhance the needling sensation. Electroacupuncture stimulation was then delivered to maintain the effects. The stimulation from this procedure was considered stronger than regular acupuncture therapy and the authors mentioned that it was important to monitor patients while performing this procedure to avoid unwanted adverse events caused by needling. The treatment duration was two weeks. Participants in the control group received medication (diclofenac sodium sustained-release tablets) for two weeks. This study reported data on the pain VAS and SF-MPQ. After the two-week treatment, all participants were followed up for another month. It was reported that the method of "stuck needle" acupuncture in combination with electroacupuncture was more effective than the medication at the end of the two-week treatment phase, and at the end of the one-month follow-up phase for pain VAS, PRI and PPI scores.

Body Acupuncture Plus Dermal Acupuncture

One study (A13) evaluated the combination of body acupuncture and dermal acupuncture, using traction therapy as the comparator. The sixty participants included in this study (30 *vs.* 30) received either acupuncture or traction therapy for two weeks. Participants in the acupuncture group first received dermal acupuncture along the Bladder meridian on the cervical and upper back region, followed by regular body acupuncture on cervical EX-B2 *Jiaji* points 颈夹脊穴, GV14 *Dazhui* 大椎, BL10 *Tianzhu* 天柱, BL11 *Dazhu* 大杼, EX-UE8 *Wai laogong* 外劳宫, and *Ashi* points 阿是穴. Both acupuncture and the traction therapy were delivered once daily. The treatment effects were assessed with the effective rate, pain VAS, SF-MPQ (total score, PRI score and PPI score) and SSCR. It was reported that after the two-week treatment, the acupuncture therapy achieved better effects than the traction therapy for all the outcome measures.

Electroacupuncture Plus Ear Acupuncture

Seventy participants were included in a study (A16) evaluating the effects of ear acupuncture plus body electroacupuncture. Acupuncture therapy was compared with traction therapy; both treatments were delivered once a day for 20 days. Participants in the acupuncture group received body electroacupuncture for 30 minutes, followed by ear acupuncture for another 30 minutes. The main body acupuncture points were: Cervical EX-B2 *Jiaji* points 颈夹脊穴, BL10 *Tianzhu* 天柱, BL11 *Dazhu* 大杼, EX-HN15 *Jing bailao* 颈百劳, and the exit of the greater occipital nerve, while the main ear acupuncture points were: AH12 *Jing* 颈, AH13 *Jingzhui* 颈椎 and SF4,5 *Jian* 肩. Individualised modifications based on Chinese medicine syndrome differentiation were also applied in terms of acupuncture points. Outcome measures were the effective rate, SF-MPQ total score, NPQ and SF-36. It was reported that the acupuncture therapy achieved significantly greater effects than the traction therapy for all outcome measures.

Assessment Using Grading of Recommendations Assessment, Development and Evaluation

The certainty of evidence for acupuncture is presented in Tables 7.4 and 7.5, with Table 7.4 presenting the certainty of evidence for acupuncture

Table 7.4. GRADE: Acupuncture *vs.* Traction Therapy

Outcome (End of Treatment)	Absolute Effect		Relative Effect (95% CI) No. of Participants (Studies)	Certainty of Evidence (GRADE)
	Acupuncture	Traction Therapy		
Effective rate	95 per 100	80 per 100	RR 1.19 (1.13, 1.25)	⊕⊕⊕◯ MODERATE[1]
	Difference: 15 more per 100 patients (95% CI: 10 more to 20 more per 100 patients)		814 (8 RCTs)	
VAS/NRS	1.90	3.14	MD −1.24 (−1.54, −0.93)	⊕⊕◯◯ LOW[1,2]
	Average difference: 1.24 lower (95% CI: 1.54 lower to 0.93 lower)		364 (5 RCTs)	
NPQ	17.45	27.58	MD −10.13 (−15.72, −4.54)	⊕⊕◯◯ LOW[1,2]
	Average difference: 10.13 lower (95% CI: 15.72 lower to 4.54 lower)		60 (1 RCT)	
MPQ PRI	3.96	6.04	MD −2.08 (−3.57, −0.6)	⊕◯◯◯ VERY LOW[1,2,3]
	Average difference: 2.08 lower (95% CI: 3.57 lower to 0.6 lower)		304 (4 RCTs)	
MPQ PPI	1.08	1.50	MD −0.42 (−0.62, −0.22)	⊕⊕◯◯ LOW[1,2]
	Average difference: 0.42 lower (95% CI: 0.62 lower to 0.22 lower)		304 (4 RCTs)	

Table 7.4.   (*Continued*)

Outcome (End of Treatment)	Absolute Effect		Relative Effect (95% CI) No. of Participants (Studies)	Certainty of Evidence (GRADE)
	Acupuncture	Traction Therapy		
MPQ total score	4.84	8.51	MD −3.67 (−5.66, −1.69)	⊕○○○ VERY
	Average difference: 3.67 lower (95% CI: 5.66 lower to 1.69 lower)		129 (2 RCTs)	LOWz[1,2,3]
SSCR	16.53	14.47	MD 20.6 (0.93, 3.19)	⊕⊕○○ LOW[1,2]
	Average difference: 2.06 higher (95% CI: 0.93 higher to 3.19 higher)		60 (1 RCT)	

The risk in the intervention group (and its 95% CI) is based on the assumed risk in the comparison group and the relative effect of the intervention (and its 95% CI).

Abbreviations: CI, confidence interval; GRADE, Grading of Recommendations Assessment, Development and Evaluation; MD, mean difference; NPQ, Northwick Park Neck Pain Questionnaire; NRS, Numeric Rating Scale; MPQ, McGill Pain Questionnaire; PPI, Present Pain Intensity; PRI, Pain Rating Index; RCT, randomised controlled trial; RR, risk ratio; SSCR, Scoring System for Cervical Radiculopathy; VAS, Visual Analogue Scale.

Notes:
1) Lack of blinding of participants and personnel may have influenced results;
2) Small sample sizes may have limited the certainty of results; and
3) High heterogeneity may have limited the certainty of results.

Study references:
Effective rate: A3, A5, A10, A12, A15, A18, A19, A21
VAS/NRS: A6, A10, A13, A15, A19
NPQ: A5
MPQ PRI: A6, A10, A13, A15
MPQ PPI: A6, A10, A13, A15
MPQ: A13, A16
SSCR: A13

in comparison with traction therapy, and Table 7.5, the certainty of the add-on effects of acupuncture to traction therapy, as below:

- Comparing acupuncture with traction therapy, the evidence of the effective rate was of "moderate" certainty, while the evidence of other outcomes was of "low" or "very low" certainty;
- Using acupuncture as an add-on therapy to traction therapy, the evidence of the effective rate and pain VAS were of "low" certainty.

Table 7.5.   GRADE: Acupuncture Plus Traction Therapy *vs.* Traction Therapy

Outcome (End of Treatment)	Absolute Effect		Relative Effect (95% CI) No. of Participants (Studies)	Certainty of Evidence (GRADE)
	Acupuncture plus Traction Therapy	Traction Therapy		
Effective rate	92 per 100	79 per 100	RR 1.17 (1.02, 1.35)	⊕⊕○○ LOW[1,2]
	Difference: 13 more per 100 patients (95% CI: 2 more to 28 more per 100 patients)		389 (5 RCTs)	
VAS/NRS	1.82	2.89	MD −1.07 (−1.35, −0.79)	⊕⊕○○ LOW[1,2]
	Average difference: 1.07 lower (95% CI: 1.35 lower to 0.79 lower)		218 (3 RCTs)	

The risk in the intervention group (and its 95% CI) is based on the assumed risk in the comparison group and the relative effect of the intervention (and its 95% CI).

Abbreviations: CI, confidence interval; GRADE, Grading of Recommendations Assessment, Development and Evaluation; MD, mean difference; NRS, Numeric Rating Scale; RCT, randomised controlled trial; RR, risk ratio; VAS, Visual Analogue Scale.

Notes:
1) Lack of blinding of participants and personnel may have influenced results;
2) Small sample sizes may have limited the certainty of results; and
3) High heterogeneity may have limited the certainty of results.

Study references:
Effective rate: A1, A4, A8, A11, A20
VAS/NRS: A1, A8, A20

Among all the evidence, the numbers of included studies and participants for most outcome measures were low (except for the effective rate), and the lack of blinding in the design of RCTs and the high heterogeneity across studies downgraded the certainty of the evidence.

Non-Controlled Studies

A total of 21 case series studies (A26–A46) were identified through our comprehensive search. A total of 1,602 patients were included in these studies. The therapies used in these studies were body acupuncture, electroacupuncture, moxibustion, warm needling, and abdominal acupuncture. Two studies (A35, A45) applied abdominal acupuncture and two studies (A27, A42) used acupuncture on the hand to treat CR.

Treatment duration ranged from six days (A35) to four weeks (A46), with 20 days being the most common duration. Chinese medicine syndrome differentiation types of patients were indicated in four studies (A27, A34, A39, A40). Of these, three studies (A27, A39, A40) explained that the common syndromes were wind-cold-dampness 风寒湿型, *qi* stagnation and Blood stasis 气滞血瘀型, and Liver-Kidney deficiency 肝肾不足型; one study (A34) applied a meridian syndrome approach to tailor treatment accordingly.

The most commonly used acupuncture points of all case series studies were: Cervical EX-B2 *Jiaji* points 颈夹脊穴 (*n* = 8) and *Ashi* points 阿是穴 (*n* = 6). Other commonly used points were: LI4 *Hegu* 合谷 (*n* = 4), GV14 *Dazhui* 大椎 (*n* = 4), BL10 *Tianzhu* 天柱 (*n* = 4), GB20 *Fengchi* 风池 (*n* = 4), and SI11 *Tianzong* 天宗 (*n* = 3).

Safety of Acupuncture Therapies

Safety information on acupuncture therapies was reported in three RCTs (A3, A19, A22) and one non-controlled study (A30). The adverse events (AEs) caused by acupuncture procedure were: (1) Five cases of slight bleeding after needle withdrawal without special concern (A3); (2) Twelve cases of subcutaneous haemorrhage after needling that were absorbed naturally (A22, A30); and (3) Four participants experiencing dizziness and nausea caused by acupuncture where the symptoms abated after resting without any additional management required (A3, A19). These participants were instructed to be better prepared before receiving acupuncture treatments and such reactions did not occur again.

All these reported AEs were mild needling events without any further medical attention needed. It could be summarised that acupuncture was safe as a treatment for CR in clinical practice.

Evidence for Acupuncture Therapies Commonly Used in Clinical Practice

A few acupuncture therapies were recommended for the management of CR, including regular body acupuncture, electroacupuncture, heat-sensitive moxibustion and ear acupressure (see Chapter 2 for details). Meta-analyses of clinical studies showed there were positive effects of overall acupuncture therapy:

- When compared with the routine care therapies in terms of the effective rate, pain VAS/NRS and MPQ scores; and
- As an add-on therapy to routine care in terms of the effective rate and pain VAS/NRS.

For specific types of acupuncture therapies, there was meta-analysis evidence supporting the following:

- Regular body acupuncture was more effective than routine care therapies for the effective rate, pain VAS/NRS, MPQ scores, and SF-36 scores;
- Adding regular body acupuncture to routine care was more effective than routine care therapies alone for the effective rate; and
- Electroacupuncture was more effective than routine care therapies for the effective rate.

GRADE assessments showed that most of the above results were of "low" or "very low" certainty.

Other types of acupuncture such as moxibustion, warm needling, "stuck needle" acupuncture 滞动针, dermal acupuncture and ear acupuncture were each evaluated by one RCT; although they all reported positive results, meta-analysis was lacking. Heat-sensitive moxibustion 热敏灸 and ear acupressure were described in Chapter 2; however, no RCTs of these therapies were included in our evaluation to show any treatment effects.

The acupuncture points used in the clinical studies were similar as those recommended in Chapter 2, where it was recommended that the principle for acupuncture point selection is choosing points in the local area (the neck and shoulder region) as the main points in combination with other distal points targeting symptoms or syndromes. Our evaluation of previously published clinical studies identified 23 RCTs and 21 non-controlled studies, and the types of acupuncture therapies used by these studies were: regular body acupuncture, electroacupuncture, moxibustion, warm needling, abdominal acupuncture, "stuck needle" acupuncture, dermal acupuncture and ear acupuncture. The most frequently used acupuncture points in these studies were all local points: Cervical EX-B2 *Jiaji* points 颈夹脊穴, GV14 *Dazhui* 大椎, *Ashi* points 阿是穴, GB20 *Fengchi* 风池 and BL10 *Tianzhu* 天柱.

Summary of Acupuncture Therapy Clinical Evidence

The evaluation of clinical studies provided certain evidence on acupuncture therapies for the treatment of CR. There are meta-analysis results and single-study results supporting the use of acupuncture therapies. However, as assessed by the GRADE approach, the certainty of most of the evidence was "low". The safety of acupuncture therapies was also evidenced, with only mild AEs caused by needling reported, but no events required any further medical management.

It is worth noting that in clinical research, acupuncture therapies were more commonly compared with routine therapies than used as add-on therapies to routine care therapies for CR. This reflects real clinical practice to a certain degree. Acupuncture therapies, in particular, regular body acupuncture and electroacupuncture, have been researched extensively. Other types of acupuncture therapy, such as moxibustion, warm needling, abdominal acupuncture, and dermal acupuncture, have also been investigated by clinical research, but there is insufficient evidence for these therapies.

Previously, there has been a considerable amount of evidence showing that acupuncture was effective for pain relief.[5–11] However, a systematic review and meta-analysis evidence on acupuncture for CR are insufficient. Our comprehensive evaluation provided meta-analysis evidence supporting the effects of overall acupuncture therapy, in particular, regular body acupuncture and electroacupuncture, in the management of CR.

As mentioned above, the most frequently used acupuncture points in all included clinical studies were all local points in the neck region. It is worth pointing out that all the RCTs evaluating electroacupuncture (*n* = 5) selected cervical EX-B2 points *Jiaji* 颈夹脊穴 (*n* = 5) in combination with other points located on relevant meridians. The EX-B2 *Jiaji* points 夹脊穴 are a group of 34 points on both sides of the spinal column, 0.5 *cun* lateral to the lower border of each spinous process, from the first thoracic vertebra to the fifth lumbar vertebra. These points can be used to treat various disorders, including those of the cardiovascular, digestive, urinary and reproductive systems. According to the Chinese medicine meridian theory, the Back-*Shu* 背俞 and EX-B2 *Jiaji* 夹脊穴 points have a relationship with the distribution of the segmental neurons of the spinal cord, and hence stimulating relevant points can regulate visceral function. Such effects can be explained as modulation of the sympathetic and parasympathetic systems.[12] Needling of EX-B2 *Jiaji* points 夹脊穴 was considered safer than needling of Back-*Shu* points 背俞穴 because perpendicular needle insertion into Back-*Shu* points 背俞穴 carries the risk of penetrating the lungs, and EX-B2 *Jiaji* points 夹脊穴 can be used as substitutes for Back-*Shu* points 背俞穴.[12] When conducting electroacupuncture on the cervical EX-B2 points *Jiaji* 颈夹脊穴 for CR, practitioners should receive proper training and ensure safety while applying electroacupuncture on these points.

The Chinese medicine syndrome differentiation approach does not play an important role in the acupuncture therapies for CR. Acupuncture point selection seems mainly focused on local points or *Ashi* points 阿是穴. Distal points were chosen in targeting other symptoms in addition to local pain. The acupuncture therapies were delivered daily or once every two days, with each acupuncture session lasting for 20 to 30 minutes. Treatment duration ranged from 10 days to four weeks, with 20 days being the most common duration. Since most of the relevant points are located on the neck, shoulder or arms, patients can receive the acupuncture treatment in a sitting position, which is helpful to reduce the time consumed for patients as well as for practitioners.

Long-term treatment effects of acupuncture were also reported by the studies, which included follow-up phases. The longest follow-up phase was six months, showing that electroacupuncture was more effective than the medication (meloxicam) in terms of the total effective rate. Other studies showed long-term effects of body acupuncture (compared with sham acupuncture), warm needling, abdominal acupuncture and "stuck needle" acupuncture compared with routine care therapies. However, there was no meta-analysis available to confirm such long-term effects.

Similar to CHM clinical research, there is inconsistency between the outcome measures reported by previously published clinical studies and those that are recommended by clinical guidelines (see Chapter 5 for more details). The effective rate was the most commonly reported outcome measure, while the NDI and SF-36 were rarely reported.

A sham control method was only used by one RCT. The lack of appropriate sham or placebo controls made it impossible to ensure the blinding of participants or acupuncture practitioners, and therefore placebo effects could not be ruled out.

References

1. 孙攀, 杜元灏, 熊俊, 黎波. (2009) 针刺与牵引治疗神经根型颈椎病疗效比较的系统评价. *光明中医* **24**(10): 1824–1830.

2. 胡进, 储浩然, 孙奎, *et al.* (2012) 针刺治疗神经根型颈椎病系统评价. *安徽中医学院学报* **31**(05): 39–43.

3. 尹逊路, 朱立国, 冯敏山, *et al.* (2018) 针刺治疗神经根型颈椎病疗效Meta分析. *康复学报* **28**(04): 63–69.

4. 薄智云. (2010) 腹针疗法[M]. 中国中医药出版社, 北京.

5. Yin C, Buchheit TE, Park JJ. (2017) Acupuncture for chronic pain: An update and critical overview. *Curr Opin Anaesthesiol* **30**(5): 583–592.

6. Linde K, Allais G, Brinkhaus B, *et al.* (2016) Acupuncture for the prevention of episodic migraine. *Cochrane Database Syst Rev* Issue 6. Art. No.: CD001218.

7. Jones L, Othman M, Dowswell T, *et al.* (2012) Pain management for women in labour: An overview of systematic reviews. *Cochrane Database Syst Rev* Issue 3. Art. No.: CD009234.

8. Zhu X, Hamilton KD, McNicol ED. (2011) Acupuncture for pain in endometriosis. *Cochrane Database Syst Rev* Issue 9. Art. No.: CD007864.

9. Linde K, Allais G, Brinkhaus B, *et al.* (2016) Acupuncture for the prevention of tension-type headache. *Cochrane Database Syst Rev* Issue 4. Art. No.: CD007587.

10. Smith CA, Collins CT, Levett KM, *et al.* (2020) Acupuncture or acupressure for pain management during labour. *Cochrane Database Syst Rev* Issue 2. Art. No.: CD009232.

11. Zhang R, Lao L, Ren K, Berman BM. (2014) Mechanisms of acupuncture–electroacupuncture on persistent pain. *Anesthesiology* **120**(2): 482–503.

12. Cabioglu MT, Arslan G. (2008) Neurophysiologic basis of Back-*shu* and *huatuo–jiaji* points. *Am J Chin Med* **36**(3): 473–479.

References to Included Clinical Studies

Study ID	Reference
A1	赵学田, 方云添, 林民辉, *et al.* (2015) 针刺后溪穴结合牵引治疗神经根型颈椎病45例临床观察. *中医药通报* **14**(1): 58–60.
A2	张红, 何立萍. (2010) 电针治疗神经根型颈椎病的临床研究. *中华全科医师杂志* **9**(3): 214–215.
A3	吴伟凡, 刘映文, 梁汉彰. (2012) 45 例神经根型颈椎病应用针灸疗法的临床比较. *中医临床研究* **4**(12): 40–41.
A4	韦衡秋, 李敏智, 陈海燕, *et al.* (2009) 中医护理干预在社区神经根型颈椎病病人康复中的应用. *护理研究* **23**(9B): 2438–2439.
A5	王莹, 沈卫东, 王文礼, *et al.* (2014) "项八针"治疗神经根型颈椎病颈痛疗效观察. *上海针灸杂志* **33**(5): 442–444.
A6	王莹, 沈卫东, 王文礼, *et al.* (2014) 用简化McGill量表评定 "项八针" 对神经根型颈椎病疼痛的影响. *针灸临床杂志* **30**(1): 7–10.
A7	王莹, 沈卫东, 王文礼. (2014) "项八针"治疗神经根型颈椎病患者生存质量的评价. *辽宁中医杂志* **41**(6): 1254–1256.
A8	刘雪芳, 汪芳, 张武昌, *et al.* (2017) 腹针配合牵引治疗神经根型颈椎病30 例. *河南中医* **37**(2): 350–352.

(*Continued*)

Study ID	Reference
A9	李波, 李建华, 吴涛. (2013) 针刺对神经根型颈椎病患者颈部肌肉表面肌电信号的影响. *中华物理医学与康复杂志* **35**(5): 395–397.
A10	陈晖阳, 谢怡琳, 杨小芬. (2015) 电针颈夹脊穴治疗神经根型颈椎病的疗效观察. *光明中医* **30**(10): 2180–2182.
A11	陈博来, 王羽丰. (2005) 牵引配合腹针治疗神经根型颈椎病 50 例疗效观察. *新中医* **37**(8): 67–68.
A12	薄智云, 牛庆强, 朱文罡, *et al.* (2005) 腹针治疗神经根型颈椎病多中心对照研究. *中国针灸* **25**(6): 387–389.
A13	晏为玮. (2016) 毫针配合皮肤针治疗神经根型颈椎病的临床疗效观察 (Thesis). 云南中医学院.
A14	吴耀持, 张峻峰, 孙懿君, *et al.* (2013) 电针治疗颈椎间盘突出症临床观察. *上海针灸杂志* **32**(12): 1035–1036.
A15	万碧江. (2006) 穴位透刺治疗神经根型颈椎病临床研究 (Thesis). 湖北中医学院.
A16	阮黄越. (2014) 电针配合耳针干预神经根型颈椎病的镇痛效应探讨 (Thesis). 南京中医药大学.
A17	乔敏, 龚广峰. (2018) 针刺治疗神经根型颈椎病的临床观察. *针灸临床杂志* **34**(01): 31–33.
A18	牛庆强. (2002) 腹针治疗神经根型颈椎病的临床疗效研究 (Thesis). 山西医科大学.
A19	陆儒. (2012) 针刺风池, 完骨, 养老, 大椎治疗神经根型颈椎病的临床研究 (Thesis). 北京中医药大学.
A20	林咸明, 罗亮, 周慧, *et al.* (2017) 颈肩同步牵引结合温针灸治疗神经根型颈椎病临床观察. *中华中医药杂志* **32**(11): 5041–5044.
A21	金载皓. (2011) 电针颈夹脊穴治疗神经根型颈椎病临床疗效观察 (Thesis). 南京中医药大学.
A22	曾正仁. (2010) 针刺颈夹脊穴治疗神经根型颈椎病的临床研究 (Thesis). 广州中医药大学.
A23	朱艳风, 韩昆, 于健, *et al.* (2018) 针刺疗法配合颈椎牵引治疗青年神经根型颈椎病的疗效观察. *心理医生* **24**(12): 135–136.
A24	邓燕琴. (2015) 滞动针配合电针疗法治疗神经根型颈椎病的临床研究 (Thesis). 广西中医药大学.
A25	Fu W-B, Liang Z-H, Zhu X-P, *et al.* (2009) Analysis on the effect of acupuncture in treating cervical spondylosis with different syndrome types. *Chin J Integr Med* **15**(6): 426–430.

(Continued)

Study ID	Reference
A26	朱伟良, 杜广中. (2014) 针刺腰阳关治疗神经根型颈椎病所致上肢酸麻胀痛13例. *中国针灸* **34**(11): 1113.
A27	朱俊. (2011) "第三掌骨疗法"治疗神经根型颈椎病 35 例. *国医论坛* **26**(1): 27.
A28	朱欢, 刘鸿燕. (2014) 恢刺法合电针治疗神经根型颈椎病 52 例疗效分析. *中医临床研究* **6**(26): 36–37.
A29	郑法文, 潘小霞. (2010) 设穴针刺治疗神经根型颈椎病 62 例效果观察. *社区医学杂志* **8**(12): 57.
A30	招文婷, 钟正, 黄泳, *et al.* (2017) 颈夹脊穴深刺导气治疗神经型颈椎病 156例临床观察. *中医药临床杂志* **29**(7): 1089–1094.
A31	张峻峰, 吴耀持. (2012) F波检测在电针治疗神经根型颈椎病疗效评价中的应用. *上海针灸杂志* **31**(12): 897–899.
A32	詹德琦. (2000) 温针灸治疗神经根型颈椎病 130 例疗效观察. *针灸临床杂志* **16**(5): 20.
A33	刘运珠. (2016) 平衡针联合经络辨证选穴治疗神经根型颈椎病 60 例. *中国针灸* **36**(8): 820.
A34	李华, 文蕾, 黄学刚. (2016) 顺经刺手三阳经郗穴为主治疗神经根型颈椎病. *中国临床医生* **44**(9): 100–101.
A35	杜健民, 王升旭, 黄泳. (2007) 薄氏腹针治疗神经根型颈椎病48例临床观察. *颈腰痛杂志* **28**(6): 531–532.
A36	周威. (2012) 经筋刺法治疗神经根型颈椎病的临床体会 (Thesis). 北京中医药大学.
A37	严全. (2015) 滞动针刺疗法治疗神经根型颈椎病 50 例(英文). *World Journal of Acupuncture-Moxibustion* **25**(02): 58–60.
A38	王雁慧, 周喜燕, 耿昌. (2005) 针刺加电针治疗神经根型颈椎病 30 例. *针灸临床杂志* **21**(07): 10.
A39	林欢熙. (2012) 梅花针与快针综合疗法治疗神经根型颈椎病（风寒湿型）的临床观察 (Thesis). 北京中医药大学.
A40	岑玉文, 杨顺益, 庄礼兴. (2000) 针灸治疗颈椎病的临床疗效观察及机理初探. *颈腰痛杂志* **21**(02): 104–107.
A41	蔡圣朝. (1996) 颈丛五针配合温灸治疗颈椎病312例疗效观察. *中国针灸* (05): 19–20.
A42	孙玉明, 刘晓清. (2001) 针刺第二掌骨全息律穴位治疗神经根型颈椎病 26 例. *安徽中医临床杂志* **13**(4): 281–282.

Study ID	Reference
A43	黄月莲. (2011) 分经辨治神经根型颈椎病 30 例. *中国针灸* **31**(9): 851–852.
A44	邓北强, 牟杨. (2018) 针刺治疗对神经根型颈椎病患者疼痛及细胞因子的影响研究. *现代医药卫生* **34**(16): 2526–2528.
A45	To J, Wang S, Huang Y. (2007) A clinical observation of Bo's abdominal acupuncture method in treating 48 cases of radiculopathic type cervical spondylosis. *Int J Clin Acupunct* **16**(2): 115.
A46	Nakajima M, Inoue M, Itoi M, *et al.* (2013) Clinical effect of acupuncture on cervical spondylotic radiculopathy: Results of a case series. *Acupunct Med* **31**(4): 364–367.

8

Clinical Evidence for Other Chinese Medicine Therapies

OVERVIEW

In addition to Chinese herbal medicine and acupuncture therapies, other Chinese medicine therapies such as cupping, *tuina* 推拿 therapy and *daoyin* 导引 exercise are commonly used clinically to manage cervical radiculopathy. This chapter provides a synopsis of the clinical trial literature and an assessment of the state of evidence.

Introduction

A rigorous screening process was undertaken to identify clinical studies of other Chinese medicine therapies for the treatment of cervical radiculopathy (CR). In addition to Chinese herbal medicine (see Chapter 5) and acupuncture therapies (see Chapter 7), other Chinese medicine therapies including *tuina* 推拿 therapy, *daoyin* 导引 exercise, cupping, etc., are also recommended by textbooks and clinical guidelines (see Chapter 2) for the management of CR. This chapter evaluates and summarises evidence of these therapies from clinical research.

Previous Systematic Reviews

Three systematic reviews were identified through our comprehensive search.[1-3] All these systematic reviews evaluated the effects of *tuina* 推拿 therapy, using conventional treatments as the comparators.

Wang *et al.*'s study in 2008 systematically reviewed RCTs and quasi-RCTs (allocation methods were not truly random) of *tuina* 推拿 therapy for CR.[1] A total of 29 studies met the selection criteria and were included in this review; 17 studies compared Chinese medicine *tuina* 推拿 therapy with traction therapy, three studies compared *tuina* 推拿 therapy with nonsteroidal anti-inflammatory drugs (NSAIDs), and nine studies compared a combination of *tuina* 推拿 therapy and traction therapy with traction therapy alone. Meta-analysis results showed: (1) In terms of the effective rate, *tuina* 推拿 therapy was more effective than NSAIDs or traction therapy, and adding *tuina* 推拿 therapy to traction therapy achieved better effects than traction therapy alone, and (2) In terms of pain Visual Analogue Scale (VAS), *tuina* 推拿 therapy was more effective than traction therapy. However, the methodological quality of most of the included trials was low, so the review authors did not draw any conclusion about *tuina* 推拿 therapy for CR.

Yang *et al.*'s study in 2013 evaluated the effects of *tuina* 推拿 therapy for CR.[2] Thirty RCTs comparing *tuina* 推拿 therapy with traction therapy were included in this review. Meta-analysis showed that *tuina* 推拿 therapy was more effective than traction therapy for the total effective rate and pain VAS at the end of the treatment phase. Long-term effects were also analysed using the outcome measure of the total effective rate, and it was found that at both the one-month post-treatment and six-month post-treatment time points, there was no difference between *tuina* 推拿 therapy and traction therapy. The authors suggested that *tuina* 推拿 therapy was effective for CR; however, it was challenging to summarise the details of the *tuina* 推拿 therapy techniques since they varied greatly across the included studies.

Wei *et al.*'s study in 2017 systematically reviewed clinical evidence of *tuina* 推拿 therapy for CR.[3] RCTs applying *tuina* 推拿 therapy alone or a combination of *tuina* 推拿 therapy and conventional treatment were evaluated. Five RCTs involving 448 patients were included in this review; of these, three RCTs compared *tuina* 推拿 therapy with cervical traction and two RCTs compared a combination of *tuina* 推拿 therapy and cervical traction with cervical traction alone. Treatment duration ranged from two to four weeks. The clinical outcome evaluated by the meta-analysis was the pain score. Meta-analysis showed that *tuina* 推拿 therapy was more effective than cervical traction, and adding *tuina* 推拿 therapy to cervical traction was more effective than cervical traction alone, for reducing pain. However, the small number and poor methodological quality of the studies weakened the evidence. The authors pointed out that there was a need for well-designed RCTs with sufficient power to confirm the effectiveness of Chinese medicine *tuina* 推拿 therapy.

Identification of Clinical Studies

A total of 20,537 citations were identified after searching Chinese databases and English databases, of which 4,369 required full-text retrieval to determine their eligibility for inclusion (Fig. 8.1). After an assessment against rigorous inclusion criteria, 70 clinical studies, which evaluated other Chinese medicine therapies for CR, were included. Forty-nine studies were RCTs (O1–O49), one (O50) was a non-randomised controlled trial and 20 (O51–O70) were non-controlled trials (Fig. 8.1). Most studies evaluated the effects of *tuina* 推拿 therapy, used alone or in combination with routine care therapies. Only two non-controlled studies (O61, O63) reported on the effect of *daoyin* 导引 exercise.

In addition, four studies evaluated therapies that are not commonly practiced outside China; these studies are not introduced in this chapter.

Randomised Controlled Trials

A total of 5,245 participants were included in the 49 RCTs (O1–O49). Participants included in these studies ranged from 18 (O38) to 69 years old (O47), with the duration of CR ranging from a day (O27) to 20 years (O13).

All the studies evaluated the effect of *tuina* 推拿 therapy for CR. The treatment duration ranged from five days (O6) to 24 weeks

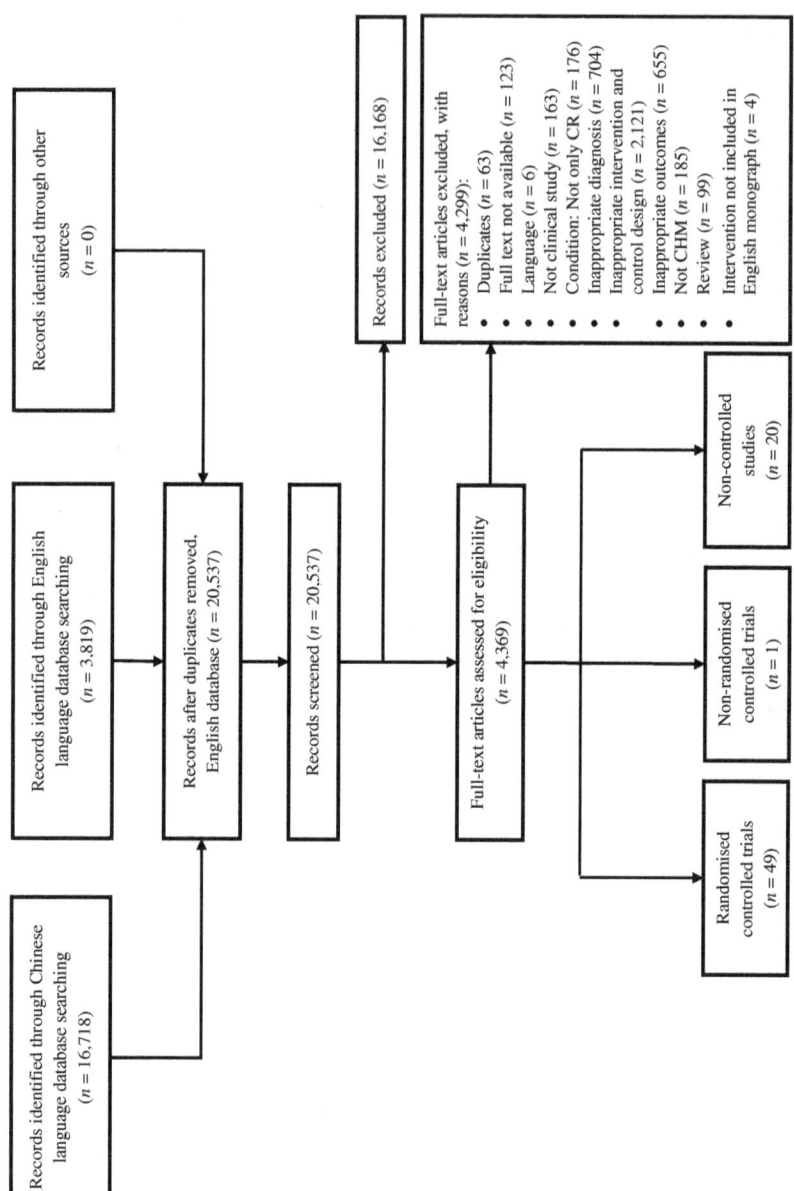

Fig. 8.1. Flow chart of the study selection process: Other Chinese medicine therapies.

(O10), with 14 days or two weeks being the most common treatment duration (O12, O14–O16, O20–O23, O25, O27–O29, O31–O33, O37, O39–O41, O44, O45, O48).

The *tuina* 推拿 therapy used by the included studies varied in terms of its specific technique. *Tuina* 推拿 therapy, also called Chinese massage, traditional Chinese massage or Chinese manipulation, is a manual therapy that includes many different types, such as acupressure, massage and "bone-setting" 正骨疗法 (orthopaedic manipulation therapy). In this monograph, *tuina* 推拿 therapy was classified into two main types: Relaxing manipulation and spinal adjusting manipulation (see Chapter 2). These two types of manipulation techniques were often applied as a combination. Thirteen RCTs (O6, O9, O12, O13, O18, O24, O26, O32, O34, O37, O38, O44, O48) applied the relaxing manipulation therapy, while the other 36 RCTs (O1–O5, O7, O8, O10, O11, O14–O17, O19–O23, O25, O27–O31, O33, O35, O36, O39–O43, O45–O47, O49) applied the spinal adjusting manipulation therapy combined with relaxing manipulation therapy.

In all included studies, 36 studies (O2–O5, O8–O16, O20, O22–O29, O31, O32, O36–O38, O40, O41, O43–O49) compared *tuina* 推拿 therapy with traction therapy, one study (O17) compared *tuina* 推拿 therapy with traction therapy plus physiotherapy, nine studies (O1, O6, O19, O21, O33–O35, O39, O42) evaluated the add-on effect of *tuina* 推拿 therapy to traction therapy, two studies (O18, O30) evaluated the add-on effect of *tuina* 推拿 therapy to traction therapy combined with physiotherapy, and one study (O7) evaluated the add-on effect of *tuina* 推拿 therapy to traction therapy combined with pharmacology therapy.

One RCT (O45) reported information on the Chinese medicine syndrome, stating that the participants included in this study were of five types: Wind-cold blocking the meridians 风寒阻络, *qi* stagnation and Blood stasis 气滞血瘀, *qi* and Blood deficiency 气血亏虚, Kidney and Liver deficiency 肝肾亏虚 and cold and dampness blocking the meridians 寒湿痹阻.

Risk-of-Bias Assessment

All included RCTs mentioned randomisation; 19 of them used appropriate methods for sequence generation, and therefore they were assessed as "low" risk of bias for this domain; the remaining studies were of "unclear" risk due to a lack of information. For allocation concealment, nine studies were at "low" risk since six of these studies applied the opaque envelope technique to conceal the participants' allocation while the other three studies applied central allocation; the remaining 40 studies were of "unclear" risk due to a lack of information.

The blinding of participants and personnel was judged as "high" risk of bias in all studies because they were all designed to compare different treatments without any effort in blinding. The blinding of outcome assessors was all at "high" risk as participants without blinding took part in the outcome assessment.

In relation to incomplete outcome data, five studies were assessed to be of "unclear" risk of bias due to a lack of information. Forty-four studies were assessed as "low" risk for not having any dropouts or a low dropout rate. Forty-seven studies without protocols were assessed as "unclear" risk for selective outcome reporting, and one study was at "high" risk since it did not report results for some of the outcomes defined in the methodology. Only one study had a published trial protocol and reported all pre-specified outcomes, so it was assessed to be of "low" risk of bias.

Overall, the methodological quality was "low" and results should be interpreted with caution. See Table 8.1 for a summary.

Outcomes

Of all predefined outcome measures (see Chapter 4), the effective rate was the most commonly reported, with it being reported in 23 studies (O1, O2, O8, O12, O13, O17, O18, O20, O21, O23, O26, O28, O29, O31, O36, O38, O39, O41–O45, O48). The pain Visual Analogue Scale (VAS) or Numeric Rating Scale (NRS) was reported by 18 studies (O1, O3, O4, O8–O10, O20, O22, O26, O31, O32,

Table 8.1. Risk-of-Bias Assessment of Randomised Controlled Trials: Other Chinese Medicine Therapies for Cervical Radiculopathy

Risk-of-Bias Domain	Low Risk n (%)	Unclear Risk n (%)	High Risk n (%)
Sequence generation	19 (38.8)	30 (61.2)	0 (0)
Allocation concealment	9 (18.4)	40 (81.6)	0 (0)
Blinding of participants	0 (0)	0 (0)	49 (100)
Blinding of personnel*	0 (0)	0 (0)	49 (100)
Blinding of outcome assessors	0 (0)	0 (0)	49 (100)
Incomplete outcome data	44 (89.8)	5 (10.2)	0 (0)
Selective outcome reporting	1 (2.0)	47 (95.9)	1 (2.0)

Note: Percentage of total randomised controlled trials (*n* = 49).

*Blinding of personnel is challenging in manual therapies.

O35, O37, O44–O46, O48, O49) and the McGill Pain Questionnaire (MPQ) by one study (O45). In terms of CR-specific outcomes, three studies (O8, O33, O46) reported data on the Neck Disability Index (NDI), three studies (O16, O39, O47) reported data on the Scoring System for Cervical Radiculopathy (SSCR), four studies (O6, O9, O10, O31) used the Assessment Scale for Cervical Spondylosis (ASCS), and four studies (O20, O23, O41, O43) used the Outcome Assessment System in the Treatment of Cervical Radiculopathy (OASTCR). In addition, one study (O46) assessed its partcipants' quality of life using the Short-Form (36) Health Survey (SF-36).

The efficacy results are presented under each comparison types and outcome as shown next.

Tuina 推拿 Therapy *vs.* Routine Care

Thirty-seven studies (O2–O5, O8–O17, O20, O22–O29, O31, O32, O36–O38, O40, O41, O43–O49) evaluated *tuina* 推拿 therapy for CR, with different routine care therapies as comparators. A total of 3,980 participants were included in these studies. Among these, 36 studies (O2–O5, O8–O16, O20, O22–O29, O31, O32, O36–O38, O40, O41, O43–O49) compared *tuina* 推拿 therapy with traction therapy and one study (O17) compared it with physiotherapy and the traction therapy. In terms of the treatment dosage, most applied the *tuina* 推拿 therapy once every two days with seven sessions in total, making it 14 days for the treatment duration. All studies used traction therapy as the comparator and most studies applied the same frequency and duration as the *tuina* 推拿 therapy.

In terms of the total effective rate, overall analysis showed that *tuina* 推拿 therapy was superior to routine care therapies (18 studies, RR: 1.17 [1.10, 1.25], $I^2 = 70\%$) (O2, O8, O12, O13, O17, O20, O23, O26, O28, O29, O31, O36, O38, O41, O43–O45, O48). Subgroup analysis also showed that *tuina* 推拿 therapy was more effective than traction therapy (17 studies, RR: 1.18 [1.00, 1.26], $I^2 = 72\%$) (O2, O8, O12, O13, O20, O23, O26, O28, O29, O31, O36, O38, O41, O43–O45, O48). In addition, one study (O17) compared *tuina* 推拿 therapy with a combination of physiotherapy and traction therapy. This study applied a kind of *tuina* 推拿 therapy called *Shi shi san bu jiu fa* 施氏三步九法, meaning "adjusting the neck in three steps using nine types of manipulation", which is a combination of relaxing manipulation therapy and spinal adjusting manipulation therapy. The results showed that this *tuina* 推拿 therapy was more effective than physiotherapy and traction therapy, improving the neck's range of motion and alleviating numbness and pain according to a self-created scale.

For the pain VAS scores, overall meta-analysis showed that *tuina* 推拿 therapy was more effective than traction therapy in relation to pain after treatment (16 studies, MD: −1.30 [−1.61, −0.99], $I^2 = 82\%$) (O3, O4, O8–O10, O20, O22, O26, O31, O32, O37, O44–O46, O48, O49).

Only one study (O45) reported data on the SF-MPQ. It showed that *tuina* 推拿 therapy was equivalent to traction therapy for the Pain Rating Index (PRI) score (MD: −1.58 [−3.21, 0.05]) or Present Pain Intensity (PPI) score (MD: −0.75 [−1.52, −0.02]). However, a superior effect was found in the VAS score.

Three studies (O8, O46, O49) reported data on the NDI and they all compared *tuina* 推拿 therapy to traction therapy, with meta-analysis showing that *tuina* 推拿 therapy was more effective than traction therapy (3 studies, MD: −6.65 [−12.52, −0.79], $I^2 = 97\%$).

Two studies (O16, O47) reported data on the SSCR, showing that there was a significant different between *tuina* 推拿 therapy and traction therapy (2 studies, MD: 3.40 [2.27, 4.54], I^2 = 71%).

Three studies (O9, O10, O31) reported data on the ASCS. Meta-analysis showed that *tuina* 推拿 therapy was more effective than traction therapy (3 studies, 3.78 [2.17, 5.40], I^2 = 72%).

For the OASTCR, overall meta-analysis showed that *tuina* 推拿 therapy was more effective than traction therapy (4 studies, MD: −4.46 [−6.70, −2.23], I^2 = 93%) (O20, O23, O41, O43).

Only one study (O46) reported data on the SF-36. A type of *tuina* 推拿 therapy called "adjusting the neck in three steps using nine types of manipulation" 整颈三步九法 was applied in this study in comparison with traction therapy. It showed there were no significant differences between the two groups in physical functioning, role-physical, bodily pain, general health, vitality, social functioning, mental health or reported health transition, but only role-emotional. This study also reported data on the NDI and pain VAS scores, showing that the *tuina* 推拿 method was more effective than traction therapy.

See Table 8.2 for a summary of the meta-analysis results.

Seven studies (O2, O4, O13, O22, O40, O44, O46) also reported data at the end of a follow-up phase. Four studies (O4, O22, O46, O49) reported data on the VAS score, with three studies (O4, O46, O49) showing the superior effects of *tuina* 推拿 therapy after a one-month follow-up phase. One study reported the VAS score at the 12- and 24-week follow-up phases, also showing the superior effects of *tuina* 推拿 therapy. One study (O22) reported the VAS data at a follow-up phase but did not mention how long the follow-up phase was.

One study (O2) assessed the effective rate and OASTCR at the end of a four-week follow-up phase; this data demonstrated the superior effects of *tuina* 推拿 therapy.

Three studies (O13, O40, O44) reported a recurrence rate, of which two studies (O13, O40) assessed the recurrence at the end of a six-month follow-up, and one study (O44) assessed it one month after treatment. All three studies showed a significant difference

Table 8.2. *Tuina* 推拿 Therapy *vs.* Routine Care Therapies

Outcome	Comparison	No. of Studies (Participants)	Effect Size (RR or MD: [95% CI], I²)	Included Studies
Effective rate	Overall: *Tuina* 推拿 therapy *vs.* routine care therapies	18 (1879)	RR: 1.17 [1.10, 1.25]*, 70%	O2, O8, O12, O13, O17, O20, O23, O26, O28, O29, O31, O36, O38, O41, O43–O45, O48
	Subgroup: *Tuina* 推拿 therapy *vs.* traction therapy	17 (1759)	RR: 1.18 [1.10, 1.26]*, 72%	O2, O8, O12, O13, O20, O23, O26, O28, O29, O31, O36, O38, O41, O43–O45, O48
VAS/NRS	Overall: *Tuina* 推拿 therapy *vs.* routine care therapies	16 (1792)	MD: −1.30 [−1.61, −0.99]*, 82%	O3, O4, O8–O10, O20, O22, O26, O31, O32, O37, O44–O46, O48, O49
NDI	Overall: *Tuina* 推拿 therapy *vs.* routine care therapies	3 (461)	MD: −6.65 [−12.52, −0.79]*, 97%	O8, O46, O49
SSCR	Overall: *Tuina* 推拿 therapy *vs.* routine care therapies	2 (199)	MD: 3.40 [2.27, 4.54]*, 71%	O16, O47
ASCS	Overall: *Tuina* 推拿 therapy *vs.* routine care therapies	3 (342)	MD: 3.78 [2.17, 5.40]*, 72%	O9, O10, O31
OASTCR	Overall: *Tuina* 推拿 therapy *vs.* routine care therapies	4 (334)	MD: −4.46 [−6.70, −2.23]*, 93%	O20, O23, O41, O43

Abbreviations: ASCS, Assessment Scale for Cervical Spondylosis; CI, confidence interval; MD, mean difference; NDI, Neck Disability Index; NRS, Numeric Rating Scale; OASTCR, Outcome Assessment System in the Treatment of Cervical Radiculopathy; RR, risk ratio; SSCR, Scoring System for Cervical Radiculopathy; VAS, Visual Analogue Scale.
*Statistically significant.

between the *tuina* 推拿 therapy group and the traction therapy group at the end of the follow-up phase. It is worth mentioning that one study (O40) reviewed the criteria for calculating the recurrence rate and suggested that a 30% increase in symptom severity should be considered "recurrence". This study also discussed the factors that may cause recurrence.

The NDI and SF-36 were assessed by two studies (O46, O49). Liu *et al.* (O40) reported data on these two outcome measures at the end of a one-month follow-up phase, showing the superior effects of *tuina* 推拿 therapy in the NDI and some domains of the SF-36. Cui *et al.* (O49) evaluated the effects of *tuina* 推拿 therapy at 2, 4, 12 and 24 weeks after randomisation. This study showed that the NDI score was lower in the *tuina* 推拿 therapy group at each time point of the follow-up phase; however, there was no significant difference in SF-36 scores.

It is worth mentioning that Cui *et al.* (O49) also reported data on a follow-up phase in the pre-protocol set (PPS) and full analysis set (FAS). This showed that the difference between the two groups was still observed in the 24-week follow-up phase for the VAS and NDI in the FAS, but disappeared in the PPS.

Tuina 推拿 Therapy Plus Routine Care Therapies *vs.* Routine Care Therapies

Twelve studies evaluated the add-on effects of other Chinese medicine therapies by comparing the combination of other Chinese medicine therapies and routine care therapies with routine care therapies alone. Nine (O1, O6, O19, O21, O33–O35, O39, O42) used traction therapy as the comparator, one study (O7) used a combination of pharmacotherapy and traction therapy and two studies (O18, O30) used a combination of physiotherapy and traction therapy as the comparator. The meta-analysis results of these studies are shown in Table 8.3.

In terms of the total effective rate, overall analysis showed that *tuina* 推拿 therapy combined with routine care therapies was superior to

Table 8.3. *Tuina* 推拿 **Therapy Plus Routine Care Therapies *vs.* Routine Care Therapies**

Outcome	Comparison	No. of Studies (Participants)	Effect Size (RR or MD: [95% CI], I²)	Included Studies
Effective rate	Overall: *Tuina* 推拿 therapy add-on to routine care therapies	10 (902)	RR: 1.07 [1.03, 1.12]*, 0%	O1, O7, O18, O19, O21, O30, O33, O34, O39, O42
	Subgroup: *Tuina* 推拿 therapy add-on to traction therapy	7 (642)	RR: 1.09 [1.04, 1.15]*, 0%	O1, O19, O21, O33, O34, O39, O42
	Subgroup: *Tuina* 推拿 therapy add-on to physiotherapy and traction therapy	2 (200)	RR: 1.07 [1.00, 1.14]*, 0%	O18, O30
VAS/NRS	Overall: *Tuina* 推拿 therapy add-on to routine care therapies	2 (198)	MD: −0.58 [−0.80, −0.37], 37%	O1, O35

Abbreviations: CI, confidence interval; NRS, Numeric Rating Scale; MD, mean difference; RR, risk ratio; VAS, Visual Analogue Scale.
*Statistically significant.

routine care therapies alone (10 studies, RR: 1.07 [1.03, 1.12], I² = 0%) (O1, O7, O18, O19, O21, O30, O33, O34, O39, O42). Subgrouping the studies according to the routine care therapies, a significant add-on benefit of *tuina* 推拿 therapy was found in the studies that used traction therapy as a comparator (7 studies, RR: 1.09 [1.04, 1.15], I² = 0%) (O1, O19, O21, O33, O34, O39, O42), as well as in the studies that used a combination of physiotherapy and traction therapy (2 studies, RR: 1.07 [1.00, 1.14], I² = 0%) (O18, O30). However, when *tuina* 推拿 therapy was added to a combination of pharmacotherapy and traction therapy, there were no add-on effects (O7).

Two studies (O1, O35) assessed the add-on effects in terms of VAS/NRS scores of *tuina* 推拿 therapy compared to traction therapy, and meta-analysis showed a significant benefit of adding *tuina* 推拿 therapy (2 studies, MD: −0.58 [−0.80, −0.37], I^2 = 37%).

Only one study (O39) reported data on the SSCR and a significant add-on benefit was found (MD: 2.62 [1.69, 3.56]).

For the ASCS, one study (O6) showed a significant add-on effect of *tuina* 推拿 therapy compared to traction therapy. This study evaluated the add-on effect of a relaxing manipulation therapy.

One study (O33) reported data on the NDI, and evaluated the add-on effect of *tuina* 推拿 therapy compared to traction therapy. It applied a spinal adjusting manipulation therapy combined with traction therapy, and the result showed that *tuina* 推拿 therapy was beneficial when added to the traction therapy.

One study (O9) reported that adding *tuina* 推拿 therapy to traction therapy was beneficial in terms of recurrence rate at the end of a six-month follow-up phase.

See Table 8.3 for a summary of the meta-analysis results.

Safety of *Tuina* 推拿 Therapy in Randomised Controlled Trials

Safety information on *tuina* 推拿 therapy was reported in 12 RCTs (O2, O7, O13, O14, O20, O29, O35, O39, O40, O43, O45, O46). Eight studies (O2, O14, O20, O39, O40, O43, O45, O46) suggested that there were no adverse events (AEs) observed. Four studies (O7, O13, O29, O35) reported that AEs occurred both in treatment groups and control groups. The AEs in the treatment groups were: (1) Two cases (O7, O35) of dizziness without special concern, (2) One case (O35) of nausea, which was relieved after resting without any treatment, (3) Seven cases of worsened pain after the *tuina* 推拿 therapy was applied, which gradually abated without any additional management required (O13, O35), and (4) Six cases of mild skin irritation, which abated naturally (O13). There were some AEs reported in control groups including nausea, dizziness, worsened pain, chest distress and mild gastrointestinal symptoms. None required any additional medical care. The other studies did not report any safety information.

Assessment Using Grading of Recommendations Assessment, Development and Evaluation

The certainty of evidence on *tuina* 推拿 therapy was assessed using GRADE and is presented in Tables 8.4 and 8.5.

Compared with traction therapy, *tuina* 推拿 therapy was superior in the aspects of the effective rate — VAS/NRS, ASCS, OASTCR and

Table 8.4.   GRADE: *Tuina* 推拿 Therapy *vs.* Traction Therapy

Outcome (End of Treatment)	Absolute Effect		Relative Effect (95% CI) No. of Participants (Studies)	Certainty of Evidence (GRADE)
	Tuina 推拿 Therapy	Traction Therapy		
Effective rate	**93** per 100	**79** per 100	**RR 1.18** (1.1, 1.26)	⊕⊕⊕◯ MODERATE[1]
	Difference: 14 more per 100 patients (95% CI: 8 more to 21 more per 100 patients)		1759 (17 RCT)	
VAS/NRS	**4.19**	**5.49**	**MD −1.30** (−1.61, −0.99)	⊕⊕◯◯ LOW[1,3]
	Average difference: 1.30 lower (95% CI: 1.61 lower to 0.99 lower)		1792 (16 RCT)	
NDI	**17.42**	**24.07**	**MD −6.65** (−12.52, −0.79)	⊕⊕◯◯ LOW[1,3]
	Average difference: 6.65 lower (95% CI: 12.52 lower to 0.79 lower)		461 (3 RCT)	
MPQ PRI	**4.11**	**5.69**	**MD −1.58** (−3.21, 0.05)	⊕⊕◯◯ LOW[1,2]
	Average difference: 1.58 lower (95% CI: 3.21 lower to 0.05 higher)		60 (1 RCT)	
MPQ PPI	**1.21**	**1.96**	**MD −0.75** (−1.52, 0.02)	⊕⊕◯◯ LOW[1,2]
	Average difference: 0.75 lower (95% CI: 1.52 lower to 0.02 higher)		60 (1 RCT)	
ASCS	**24.26**	**20.48**	**MD 3.78** (2.17, 5.4)	⊕⊕◯◯ LOW[1,2]
	Average difference: 3.78 higher (95% CI: 2.17 higher to 5.4 higher)		342 (3 RCT)	

Table 8.4. (*Continued*)

Outcome (End of Treatment)	Absolute Effect		Relative Effect (95% CI) No. of Participants (Studies)	Certainty of Evidence (GRADE)
	Tuina 推拿 Therapy	Traction Therapy		
OASTCR	5.96	10.42	MD −4.46 (−6.70, −2.23)	⊕○○○ VERY LOW[1,2,3]
	Average difference: 4.46 lower (95% CI: 6.70 lower to 2.23 lower)		334 (4 RCT)	
SSCR	19.46	16.06	MD 3.40 (2.27, 4.54)	⊕⊕○○ LOW[1,2]
	Average difference: 3.40 higher (95% CI: 2.27 higher to 4.54 higher)		199 (2 RCT)	

The risk in the intervention group (and its 95% CI) is based on the assumed risk in the comparison group and the relative effect of the intervention (and its 95% CI).

Abbreviations: ASCS, Assessment Scale for Cervical Spondylosis; CI, confidence interval; GRADE, Grading of Recommendations Assessment, Development and Evaluation; MD, mean difference; NDI, Neck Disability Index; NRS, Numeric Rating Scale; MPQ, McGill Pain Questionnaire; OASTCR, Outcome Assessment System in the Treatment of Cervical Radiculopathy; PPI, Present Pain Intensity; PRI, Pain Rating Index; RCT, randomised controlled trial; RR, risk ratio; SSCR, Scoring System for Cervical Radiculopathy; VAS, Visual Analogue Scale.

Notes:
1) Lack of blinding of participants and personnel may have influenced results;
2) Small sample size may have limited the certainty of results; and
3) High heterogeneity may have limited the certainty of results.

Study references:
Effective rate: O2, O8, O12, O13, O17, O20, O23, O26, O28, O29, O31, O36, O38, O41, O43–O45, O48
VAS/NRS: O3, O4, O8–O10, O20, O22, O26, O31, O32, O37, O44–O46, O48, O49
NDI: O8, O46, O49
MPQ PRI: O45
MPQ PPI: O45
ASCS: O9, O10, O31
OASTCR: O20, O23, O41, O43
SSCR: O16, O47

SSCR — but there were no significant differences between *tuina* 推拿 therapy and traction therapy in PPI or PRI. The certainty of this evidence was assessed as "very low", "low" or "moderate" (Table 8.4).

Table 8.5. GRADE: *Tuina* 推拿 Therapy Plus Traction Therapy *vs.* Traction Therapy

Outcome (End of Treatment)	Absolute Effect		Relative Effect (95% CI) No. of Participants (Studies)	Certainty of Evidence (GRADE)
	Tuina 推拿 Therapy plus Traction Therapy	Traction Therapy		
Effective rate	**93** per 100	**85** per 100	**RR 1.09** (1.04, 1.15)	⊕⊕⊕◯ MODERATE[1]
	Difference: 8 more per 100 patients (95% CI: 3 more to 13 more per 100 patients)		642 (7 RCT)	
VAS/NRS	**1.68**	**2.26**	**MD −0.58** (−0.80, −0.37)	⊕⊕◯◯ LOW[1,2]
	Average difference: 0.58 lower (95% CI: 0.80 lower to 0.37 lower)		198 (2 RCT)	
NDI	**9.25**	**11.37**	**MD −2.12** (−2.83, −1.41)	⊕⊕◯◯ LOW[1,2]
	Average difference: 2.12 lower (95% CI: 2.83 lower to 1.41 lower)		60 (1 RCT)	
ASCS	**25.83**	**22.00**	**MD 3.83** (2.64, 5.02)	⊕⊕◯◯ LOW[1,2]
	Average difference: 3.83 higher (95% CI: 2.64 higher to 5.02 higher)		72 (1 RCT)	
SSCR	**17.86**	**15.24**	**MD 2.62** (1.69, 3.56)	⊕⊕◯◯ LOW[1,2]
	Average difference: 2.62 higher (95% CI: 1.69 higher to 3.56 higher)		90 (1 RCT)	

The risk in the intervention group (and its 95% CI) is based on the assumed risk in the comparison group and the relative effect of the intervention (and its 95% CI).

Abbreviations: ASCS, Assessment Scale for Cervical Spondylosis; CHM, Chinese herbal medicine; CI, confidence interval; GRADE, Grading of Recommendations Assessment, Development and Evaluation; MD, mean difference; NDI, Neck Disability Index; NRS, Numeric Rating Scale; RCT, randomised controlled trial; RR, risk ratio; SSCR, Scoring System of Cervical Radiculopathy; VAS, Visual Analogue Scale.

Notes:
1) Lack of blinding of participants and personnel may have influenced results;
2) Small sample size may have limited the certainty of results; and
3) High heterogeneity may have limited the certainty of results.

Study references:
Effective rate: O1, O19, O21, O33, O34, O39, O42
VAS/NRS: O1, O35
NDI: O33
ASCS: O6
SSCR: O39

When *tuina* 推拿 therapy was used as an add-on to traction therapy, it was found to be beneficial in terms of the effective rate — VAS/NRS, NDI, ASCS and SSCR. This evidence was assessed to be of "moderate" or "low" certainty (Table 8.5).

Clinicians should consider this when selecting *tuina* 推拿 therapy for the treatment of CR.

Non-Randomised Controlled Trials

One non-randomised controlled trial (O50) compared *tuina* 推拿 to traction therapy on 106 patients. The *tuina* 推拿 therapy used in this study was a combination of spinal adjusting manipulation and the relaxing manipulation therapy. The treatment duration was two weeks. The effective rate was used to assess the treatment effects, showing that *tuina* 推拿 therapy was more effective than traction therapy. The safety information was not reported.

Non-Controlled Studies

Twenty non-controlled case series studies (O51–O70) reported the effects of other Chinese medicine therapies for CR. A total of 1,752 patients were included in these studies. The therapies used in these studies were *tuina* 推拿 therapy and *daoyin* 导引 exercise. Six studies (O52, O57, O64, O65, O69, O70) only applied a relaxing manipulation therapy, 12 studies (O51, O53–O56, O58–O60, O62, O66–O68) applied the spinal adjusting manipulation therapy combined with relaxing manipulation therapy and two studies (O61, O63) applied *daoyin* 导引 exercise.

The treatment duration of the *tuina* 推拿 therapy ranged from 10 days (O56, O60) to 30 days (O62), with 14 days being the most common duration (O51, O54, O57, O58). The treatment frequency of *tuina* 推拿 therapy was either once a day or three times a week. *Daoyin* 导引 exercise is a type of gentle exercise practised by patients themselves; its duration ranged from 30 days (O61) to 12 weeks (O63) and the frequency ranged from twice per day to twice per week. One study (O52) reported Chinese medicine syndrome differentiation types of patients. The outcomes reported by these studies were the effective rate ($n = 20$) (O51–O70), VAS ($n = 2$) (O52, O63), OASTCR ($n = 2$) (O54, O58) and ASCS ($n = 1$) (O63).

It was worth noting that three studies (O51, O58, O67) applied a specific type of *tuina* 推拿 therapy, namely *shuchun sun* manipulation. These studies reported data on its effective rate and OASTCR.

Two studies (O61, O63) applied *daoyin* 导引 exercises; these were *tai chi zen cloud-like moving hands* 太极禅云手 and *Shi's twelve-word exercise* 施氏十二字养生功. Guo *et al.* (O63) reported the effect of *tai chi zen cloud-like moving hands* 太极禅云手 for CR. This study was a prospective case series with 139 patients involved. *Tai chi zen cloud-like moving hands* 太极禅云手 was applied twice a week, 150 minutes each time from the first to the fourth week, then 60 minutes each time from the fifth to the twelfth week. The VAS and a self-created scale were reported as the outcome measures. Jia *et al.* (O61) reported clinical research on *Shi's twelve-word exercise* 施氏十二字养生功 for CR; this exercise was applied twice a day for 30 days as one session. The results were assessed after two sessions, using a self-created scale as the outcome measure.

Safety of Other Chinese Medicine Therapies in Non-Controlled Studies

Safety information was mentioned in two studies (O65, O62) on 140 participants, one (O65) reporting that there were no AEs during the treatment phase and the other study (O62) reporting AEs including paleness, dizziness, sweatiness, nausea and worsened pain. All these AEs were mild events without any further medical attention needed.

Evidence for Other Chinese Medicine Therapies Commonly Used in Clinical Practice

Cupping therapy, *tuina* 推拿 therapy and *daoyin* 导引 exercise are recommended by clinical guidelines for the treatment of CR (see Chapter 2).

There were three previously published systematic reviews of other Chinese medicine therapies for CR identified in our comprehensive search. All of them evaluated the *tuina* 推拿 therapy, but most of the included trials had a high risk of bias, so the three reviews did not draw any conclusion on the *tuina* 推拿 therapy for CR.

No clinical evidence of the cupping therapy was found in our research. This could be explained by the predefined inclusion criteria of this research which prevented the inclusion of clinical studies on cupping. There is a need for clinical research on the cupping therapy following a rigorous methodology.

Most of the included studies (*n* = 68) applied *tuina* 推拿 therapy for CR, including all RCTs, one CCT and 18 non-controlled studies. Thirty-six RCTs and one CCT compared *tuina* 推拿 therapy with traction therapy and one RCT compared it with physiotherapy and traction therapy. Nine studies evaluated the add-on effect of *tuina* 推拿 therapy to traction therapy, one study evaluated the add-on effect of *tuina* 推拿 therapy to pharmacotherapy and traction therapy, and two studies evaluated it in relation to physiotherapy and traction therapy.

There are two types of *tuina* 推拿 therapy, as mentioned in Chapter 2 — relaxing manipulation therapy and spinal adjusting mani-pulation therapy. Of all the included studies, 17 studies applied the relaxing manipulation therapy and 51 applied the spinal adjusting manipulation therapy combined with a relaxing manipulation therapy. This shows that both these styles of therapy are commonly used in China.

Among the 17 studies that applied the relaxing manipulation therapy, 12 studies were RCTs and five studies were non-controlled. Twelve RCTs applied traction therapy as the comparator, using the effective rate — VAS/NRS, ASCS and SF-36 — as outcome measures. The meta-analysis showed that the relaxing manipulation therapy was more effective than traction therapy in terms of the pain VAS, but no different to the traction therapy assessed by the effective rate. The five non-controlled studies used the effective rate as the outcome measure. The results for the effective rate were above 91.3% in each study, indicating a satisfactory treatment effect.

On the other hand, among the 51 studies that applied the spinal adjusting manipulation therapy combined with a relaxing manipulation therapy, 37 studies were RCTs, one study was a non-randomised controlled trial and 13 studies were non-controlled. Twenty-seven RCTs applied traction therapy as the comparator and one RCT used traction therapy and physiotherapy as the comparator. Seven RCTs evaluated the add-on effect of the combination manipulation therapy to traction therapy, one RCT evaluated the add-on effect to traction therapy and physiotherapy, and one RCT evaluated the add-on effect to traction therapy and pharmacology therapy. They used the effective rate — VAS/NRS, MPQ, NDI, ASCS, SSCR, OASTCR and SF-36 — as outcome measures. The meta-analysis showed that the combination manipulation therapy was superior to traction therapy when using the effective rate and VAS as outcome measures. The result of one non-randomised controlled trial showed that the combination manipulation therapy was more effective than traction therapy. The 13 non-controlled studies used the effective rate as the outcome measure. These were above 90% in each study, indicating a satisfactory treatment effect.

In sum, the overall effect of *tuina* 推拿 therapy for CR is promising. Only two non-controlled studies evaluated *daoyin* 导引 exercise. The effects of *tai chi zen cloud-like moving hands* 太极禅云手 and *Shi's twelve-word exercise* 施氏十二字养生功 were assessed by these studies and it was reported that *daoyin* 导引 exercise could be considered a low-cost, low-risk and effective therapy for CR. Only four studies (O38, O42, O45, O52) mentioned treatment based on syndrome differentiation. The main types of syndrome were wind and cold blocking meridians 风寒阻络, and *qi* stagnation and Blood stasis 气滞血瘀.

Summary of Other Chinese Medicine Therapies Clinical Evidence

This chapter evaluated the effect of other Chinese medicine therapies for CR. A total of 70 studies met the inclusion criteria, including 68 studies that applied *tuina* 推拿 therapy and two studies that applied *daoyin* 导引 exercise.

The cupping therapy was not evaluated by the studies included in our research.

Our review of clinical studies found that *tuina* 推拿 therapy was beneficial for CR as suggested by the meta-analyses:

- *Tuina* 推拿 therapy was more effective than routine care therapies in terms of the effective rate (meta-analysis of 18 RCTs), VAS (meta-analysis of 16 RCTs), NDI (meta-analysis of three RCTs), SSCR (meta-analysis of two RCTs), ASCS (meta-analysis of three RCTs) and OASTCR (meta-analysis of four RCTs); and
- *Tuina* 推拿 therapy plus routine care therapies were more effective than routine care therapies alone in terms of the effective rate (meta-analysis of 10 RCTs), pain VAS/NRS (meta-analysis of two RCTs), ASCS (one RCT), SSCR (one RCT) and NDI (one RCT).

The treatment duration of *tuina* 推拿 therapy ranged from five days to 24 weeks, with 14 days or two weeks being the most common treatment duration. *Tuina* 推拿 therapy was conducted once a day or once every two days, and usually consisted of 20 to 30 minutes for each session.

The meta-analysis showed that two types of *tuina* 推拿 therapy — relaxing manipulation therapy and spinal adjusting manipulation therapy — were both significantly effective for CR. The relaxing manipulation therapy could be applied alone or combined with the spinal adjusting manipulation therapy.

However, as the GRADE assessment showed that the certainty of the clinical evidence on *tuina* 推拿 therapy was "moderate", "low" or "very low", the interpretation and clinical application of these therapies should be done with caution. Nevertheless, more evidence is needed to confirm the effects of these therapies.

In terms of long-term effects, eight studies reported data on a follow-up phase. It seems that the *tuina* 推拿 therapy could relieve the symptoms of CR in the short term compared to the traction therapy, but the long-term effects were not superior to those of the traction therapy. In addition, based on the data from three studies, it seems that the *tuina* 推拿 therapy could reduce the recurrence rate.

With regard to the safety of *tuina* 推拿 therapy, there were no severe AEs reported by the included clinical studies, though there were some mild symptoms without any additional medical care needed in five studies (four RCTs, one non-controlled study), including gastrointestinal symptoms, pain and skin irritation. Furthermore, due to the lack of long-term follow-up in most studies, it was not possible to find out whether there were any delayed noticeable AEs from the *tuina* 推拿 therapy.

Two non-controlled studies applied *daoyin* 导引 exercises. The results showed that *daoyin* 导引 exercise was beneficial for CR for the pain VAS, ASCS and a self-created scale. There was no safety information about *daoyin* 导引 exercises reported, but according to the nature of this exercise, it could be considered a low-risk, low-cost therapy that would be easy to fit into patients' daily activities.

In summary, there is some evidence supporting the use of other Chinese medicine therapies for CR, especially *tuina* 推拿 therapy. Although the detailed techniques of these therapies varied, it is suggested that the *tuina* 推拿 therapy could be applied once every two days for a total of seven sessions, since this is the most common frequency in the included studies.

References

1. 王宾. (2011) 手法治疗神经根型颈椎病随机对照试验的系统评价及施治规律探讨 (Thesis). 北京中医药大学.
2. 杨佳, 张瑞春, 王新军. (2013) 推拿与牵引治疗神经根型颈椎病的 Meta 分析. *环球中医药* **6**(9): 641–648.
3. Wei X, Wang S, Li L, Zhu L. (2017) Clinical evidence of Chinese massage therapy (*tui na*) for cervical radiculopathy: A systematic review and meta-analysis. *Evid Based Complement Alternat Med* **2017**(9): 1–10.

References to Included Clinical Studies

O1 竺永达, 李石胜. (2015) 手法推拿结合牵引治疗神经根型颈椎病的临床观察. *现代实用医学* **27**(5): 673–675.

O2 朱立国, 张清, 高景华, *et al.* (2005) 旋转手法治疗神经根型颈椎病的临床观察. *中国骨伤* **18**(8): 489–490.

O3 朱立国, 于杰, 高景华, *et al.* (2005) 旋转手法治疗神经根型颈椎病对疼痛的 vas 评分临床研究 *北京中医* **24**(5): 297–298.

O4 朱立国, 于杰, 高景华, *et al.* (2009) 神经根型颈椎病患者的疼痛和麻木观测. *中国中医骨伤科杂志* **17**(4): 1–3.

O5 朱国苗. (2012) 旋转拔伸手法治疗神经根型颈椎病的临床经济学研究. *时珍国医国药* **23**(9): 2338–2339.

O6 周晶, 吴淼, 郝建波. (2014) 开返魂锁辅助治疗社区神经根型颈椎病的疗效观察及应用推广. *湖北中医药大学学报* **16**(2): 72–74.

O7 周宾宾, 韦坚, 韦贵康. (2008) 侧旋提推手法治疗神经根型颈椎病疗效观察. *中医正骨* **20**(10): 8–9.

O8 赵岩, 史晓林. (2012) 整颈三步九法治疗神经根型颈椎病疗效观察. *浙江中医药大学学报* **36**(11): 1225–1227, 1230.

O9 章家福, 林强, 苑洁. (2011) 推拿治疗青年期神经根型颈椎病的随机对照研究. *针灸推拿医学·英文版* **9**(4): 249–252.

O10 张盼, 杨明. (2017) 三小定点整脊术治疗神经根型颈椎病 73 例临床观察. *湖南中医杂志* **33**(10): 94–96.

O11 张明才, 石印玉, 陈东煜, *et al.* (2011) 矫正关节突关节"骨错缝"手法治疗神经根型颈椎病的有效性研究. *上海中医药杂志* **45**(12): 42–45.

O12 张成, 齐伟. (2014) 定点牵伸法治疗神经根型颈椎病 60 例. *长春中医药大学学报* **30**(2): 327–328.

O13 詹红生, 牛守国, 吴健康, *et al.* (2006) 仰卧位拔伸整复手法治疗神经根型颈椎病的随机, 对照, 多中心临床研究. *中国骨伤* **19**(5): 257–260.

O14 俞乐, 陈红蕾, 林伟锋. (2008) 定位整复手法治疗神经根型颈椎病 60 例. *江西中医药* **39**(4): 36–37.

O15 于嘉, 谢雁鸣, 朱立国, *et al.* (2008) 旋转手法治疗神经根型颈椎病成本效果分析. *中国中医药信息杂志* **15**(4): 7–8.

O16 殷华俊, 王剑, 白晶, *et al.* (2014) 仰卧位定点扳法治疗神经根型颈椎病 50 例. *中国中医药现代远程教育* **12**(2): 39–40.

O17 叶秀兰, 唐占英, 钱雪华, *et al.* (2008) 施氏三步九法治疗神经根型颈椎病临床研究. *上海中医药杂志* **42**(5): 51–53.

(Continued)

(*Continued*)

O18 徐鑫亚. (2011) 推拿配合牵引超短波在治疗神经根型颈椎病中的作用. *按摩与康复医学* **2**(36): 56.

O19 吴翔, 刘福水. (2007) 正骨推拿手法配合牵引治疗神经根型颈椎病疗效观察. *按摩与导引* **23**(1): 2–3, 11.

O20 王乾, 朱立国, 高景华, *et al.* (2009) 旋提手法治疗神经根型颈椎病的疗效观察. *中医正骨* **21**(6): 9–11.

O21 王军涛, 张文骞, 邹亮. (2015) 卧位牵顿手法治疗神经根型颈椎病临床研究. *山东中医杂志* **34**(4): 264–266.

O22 王红东, 李俊杰, 刘克新, *et al.* (2010) 旋提手法治疗神经根型颈椎病观察. *世界中医骨科杂志* **11**(2): 87–89.

O23 孙武权, 谢贤斐, 王佳勤, *et al.* (2010) 脊柱微调手法治疗神经根型颈椎病疗效与颈椎曲度变化观察. *中华中医药杂志* **25**(9): 1526–1528.

O24 隋广馨, 马玉祺, 李智. (2009) 卧位整复手法治疗神经根型颈椎病 60 例临床观察. *江苏中医药* **41**(5): 52–53.

O25 秦毅, 李振宇, 鲁尧, *et al.* (2012) 孙氏旋转手法治疗神经根型颈椎病临床研究. *中国中医骨伤科杂志* **20**(7): 3–5.

O26 米仲祥, 毕军伟. (2013) 推拿治疗神经根型颈椎病的临床疗效观察. *西部中医药* **26**(7): 101–102.

O27 刘鹏, 李远栋, 张君涛, *et al.* (2011) 旋提手法对神经根型颈椎病曲度改变的疗效分析. *天津中医药* **28**(4): 298–300.

O28 刘鹏, 李层, 马晓飞. (2015) 定点拔升旋转复位法治疗神经根型颈椎病的疗效观察. *湖北中医杂志* **37**(12): 66–67.

O29 林远方, 朱其广, 郑晓斌, *et al.* (2011) 卧位牵顿手法治疗神经根型颈椎病临床研究. *中国中医骨伤科杂志* **19**(12): 14–16.

O30 林景琳, 杨锦玲. (2004) 旋转复位与牵引治疗神经根型颈椎病的随机对照疗效分析. *中国临床康复* **8**(17): 3234–3235.

O31 黎顺平, 唐上德, 王云娜, *et al.* (2017) 尚德正骨手法治疗中青年神经根型颈椎病40例. *山东中医杂志* **36**(10): 876–878.

O32 蒋崇博, 王军, 郑志新, *et al.* (2012) 颈椎定点引伸手法治疗神经根型颈椎病的随机对照研究. *中西医结合学报* **10**(1): 54–58.

O33 贾江波, 杜海峡. (2017) 颈项旋扳法结合颈椎牵引治疗神经根型颈椎病 30 例. *中国民族民间医药杂志* **26**(24): 88–89.

O34 黄振俊, 陈建新. (2010) 五步手法配合牵引治疗神经根型颈椎病的临床研究. *中医学报* **25**(5): 1012–1013.

(*Continued*)

O35 胡文杰, 李阳, 王涛, *et al.* (2018) 拔伸旋转整脊手法联合颈椎牵引治疗神经根型颈椎病临床观察. *河北中医* **40**(4): 593–595, 618.

O36 高国栋, 张晓刚, 宋敏, *et al.* (2012) "三步二位五法"治疗神经根型颈椎病150 例临床观察. *中国中医骨伤科杂志* **20**(4): 18–20.

O37 范京强, 郭程湘, 陈博来, *et al.* (2011) 郭氏"畅气通络"手法治疗神经根型颈椎病的疗效观察. *实用医学杂志* **27**(12): 2267–2269.

O38 赵可心. (2010) 点按法治疗神经根型颈椎病的临床研究 (Thesis). 长春中医药大学.

O39 张文远. (2014) 牵引下正骨法治疗神经根型颈椎病的临床研究 (Thesis). 长春中医药大学.

O40 于杰. (2010) 神经根型颈椎病复发及相关因素的临床研究 (Thesis). 中国中医科学院.

O41 于嘉. (2006) 旋转手法治疗神经根型颈椎病临床疗效评价和成本 —— 效果分析 (Thesis). 中国中医科学院.

O42 王海亮. (2010) 推拿配合牵引治疗神经根型颈椎病的临床研究 (Thesis). 长春中医药大学.

O43 孟庆楠. (2010) 旋转手法治疗神经根型颈椎病的临床研究 (Thesis). 长春中医药大学.

O44 李玉斌. (2010) 屈颈正骨手法治疗神经根型颈椎病的临床研究 (Thesis). 湖北中医药大学.

O45 李锐涛. (2012) 龙氏正骨推拿治疗神经根型颈椎病的临床研究 (Thesis). 广州中医药大学.

O46 刘华. (2013) 整颈三步九法治疗神经根型颈椎病临床观察 (Thesis). 河南中医药大学.

O47 李普光. (2002) 孙氏手法治疗神经根型颈椎病的临床和实验研究 (Thesis). 中国中医科学院骨伤科研究所; 中国中医科学院; 中国中医研究院骨伤科研究所.

O48 蒋崇博. (2012) 王军教授治疗脊柱相关性疾病软组织疼痛手法经验研究 (Thesis). 解放军总医院; 解放军医学院; 军医进修学院; 军医进修学院解放军总医院.

O49 Cui X-J, Yao M, Ye X-L, *et al.* (2017) Shi-style cervical manipulations for cervical radiculopathy: A multicenter randomized-controlled clinical trial. *Medicine* **96**(31): e7276.

O50 王少伟, 李伟居, 黄桂忠. (2007) 动点定位旋扳手法治疗神经根型颈椎病的临床观察. *中国中医骨伤科杂志* **15**(4): 47–49.

(Continued)

(Continued)

O51 朱峥嵘. (2008) 手法治疗神经根型颈椎病 61 例. *中国中医急症* **17**(5): 697–698.

O52 杨功旭, 王胜利, 方苏亭, *et al.* (2009) 点揉补泻手法治疗颈神经根炎临床研究. *中国中医骨伤科杂志* **17**(3): 32–33.

O53 王洋, 宋哲, 刘硕. (2009) 神经根型颈椎病 102 例按摩治疗体会. *临床误诊误治* **22**(5): 19–20.

O54 王琼, 朱国苗. (2013) 旋转拔伸手法治疗神经根型颈椎病的疗效与颈椎 x 线的 logistic 回归分析研究. *颈腰痛杂志* **34**(6): 452–455.

O55 覃飞. (2011) 牵引加手法治疗青少年神经根型颈椎病 50 例. *陕西中医* **32**(4): 436–438.

O56 苏良喜, 翁文水, 王小燕. (2012) "短杠杆微调"手法治疗神经根型颈椎病 63 例疗效观察. *按摩与康复医学* **3**(1): 57–59.

O57 宋郁如, 吕智桢, 吕立江, *et al.* (2011) 仰卧牵枕法治疗神经根型颈椎病的临床观察. *中医临床研究* **3**(23): 26–27.

O58 宋永伟. (2011) 应用孙氏旋提手法治疗神经根型颈椎病. *中医正骨* **23**(4): 67–68.

O59 李正祥. (2010) 脊柱微调手法治疗神经根型颈椎病 137 例. *山东中医杂志* **29**(6): 392–393.

O60 李新建. (2013) 推拿治疗神经根型颈椎病的临床疗效观察. *按摩与康复医学* **4**(3): 67–68.

O61 贾宽, 李旭东, 孙爱军, *et al.* (2014) 施氏十二字养生功对社区神经根型颈椎病患者康复效果观察. *长春中医药大学学报* **30**(4): 695–697.

O62 黄永. (2006) 综合治疗神经根型颈椎病 120 例. *湖南中医杂志* **22**(5): 31–32.

O63 郭姜, 王得志, 闵萧, *et al.* (2018) 太极禅云手防治神经根型颈椎病临床综合评价研究. *中华中医药杂志* **33**(3): 1198–1200.

O64 陈滢华, 徐联洋, 彭旭明. (2015) 推拿治疗神经根型颈椎病 120 例疗效观察. *按摩与康复医学* **6**(17): 48–49.

O65 李书纳. (2014) 拔伸旋转手法对神经根型颈椎病肌电图变化的影响 (Thesis). 河南中医学院.

O66 姜贵云. (1988) 推拿治疗神经根型颈椎病 104 例疗效观察. *承德医学院学报* **5**(03): 164–165, 187.

O67 钟康华, 陈仕梅, 肖懔祺, *et al.* (2012) 孙氏手法治疗神经根型颈椎病的疗效观察. *按摩与康复医学* **3**(4): 63–64.

(*Continued*)

O68	苏霄乐, 翁文水, 罗晓英. (2013) 丁季峰(扌衮)法配合被动运动治疗神经根型颈椎病疗效观察. *光明中医* **28**(5): 896–897.
O69	刘克龙. (2010) 推拿配合手法牵引治疗神经根型颈椎病. *中国民间疗法* **18**(10): 27.
O70	鲍建飞. (2017) 五线五区十三穴推拿法治疗神经根型颈椎病. *内蒙古中医药* **16**: 109.

9

Clinical Evidence for Chinese Medicine Combination Therapy

OVERVIEW

A combination of different types of Chinese medicine therapies is commonly used in clinical practice for the management of cervical radiculopathy. This chapter evaluates the evidence from clinical studies which used Chinese medicine combination therapy for this condition.

Introduction

This chapter evaluates the clinical evidence for using combinations of different types of Chinese medicine therapies to treat cervical radiculopathy (CR). Studies combining the same type of Chinese medicine therapies have been presented in Chapter 5 (e.g., oral and topical Chinese herbal medicine [CHM]), Chapter 7 (e.g., body acupuncture and ear acupuncture) and Chapter 8 (e.g., *tuina* 推拿 therapy plus *daoyin* 导引 exercise). In clinical practice, applying a combination of more than one type of Chinese medicine therapy is very common, although it is difficult for clinical researchers to identify the efficacy of each therapy used in these combinations. The treatment effects of Chinese medicine combination therapy are presented in this chapter under each combination.

Previous Systematic Reviews

Our comprehensive search did not identify any previous systematic review that meets the selection criteria.

Identification of Clinical Studies

A search of nine English- and Chinese-language databases identified 20,537 citations, of which 4,369 required full-text retrieval to determine their eligibility for inclusion (Fig. 9.1). After an assessment against rigorous inclusion criteria, 18 randomised controlled trials (RCTs) (C1–C18) and 38 non-controlled studies (C19–C56) were included in our evaluation. In addition, ten studies applied Chinese medicine therapies which are not commonly practised outside China; these studies are not discussed in this chapter.

Randomised Controlled Trials

Eighteen RCTs (C1–C18) investigated the effects of Chinese medicine combination therapy for the treatment of CR. One study (C16) was published in English, and the other 17 studies were published in Chinese. A total of 3,135 participants were involved in these studies. Participants ranged from 18 (C1) to 65 years (14), with the duration of CR ranging from one week (C12) to 23 years (C12).

The Chinese medicine therapies evaluated by the included RCTs were: CHM, acupuncture, cupping, *tuina* 推拿 therapy and *daoyin* 导引 exercise. These therapies were applied as combinations of two or three therapies, as shown in Table 9.1. Four RCTs (C1, C2, C10, C17) evaluated the add-on effects of Chinese medicine combination therapy to routine care therapies, and the other RCTs compared Chinese medicine therapies in combination with routine care therapies, including pharmacotherapy, traction therapy and physiotherapy, or their combinations.

The treatment duration ranged from two weeks (C3, C5–C9, C13–C15) to 25 days (C17), with two weeks being the most common treatment duration. One RCT (C3) reported information on Chinese medicine syndrome differentiation; it was reported that patients with CR had phlegm and dampness blocking meridians, Liver and Kidney deficiency, *qi* and Blood deficiency, and *qi* stagnation and Blood deficiency (痰湿阻络, 肝肾不足, 气血亏虚, 气滞血瘀).

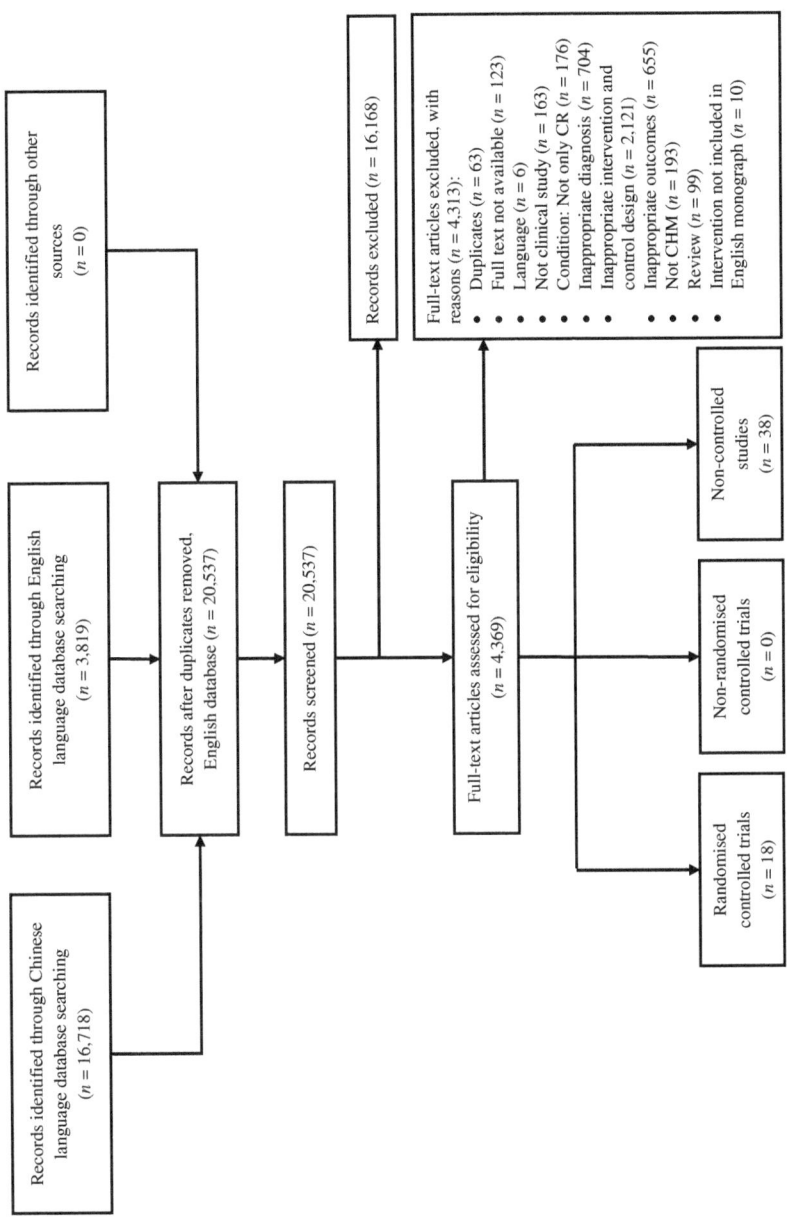

Fig. 9.1. Flow chart of the study selection process: Chinese medicine combination therapy.

229

Table 9.1. Summary of Interventions in Chinese Medicine Combination Therapy Studies

Chinese Medicine Combination Studies	No. of Studies	Included Studies
CHM and acupuncture	2	C8, C10
CHM and *tuina* 推拿 therapy	3	C3, C11, C14
CHM and *tuina* 推拿 therapy and *daoyin* 导引 exercise	4	C5, C6, C13, C15
Acupuncture and *tuina* 推拿 therapy	4	C4, C7, C9, C18
Acupuncture and cupping	2	C12, C16
Acupuncture and *daoyin* 导引 exercise	1	C1
Acupuncture and *tuina* 推拿 therapy and *daoyin* 导引 exercise	2	C2, C17

Abbreviation: CHM, Chinese herbal medicine.

Nine RCTs (C3, C5, C6, C8, C10, C11, C13–C15) evaluated the combination of CHM and other Chinese medicine therapies. One RCT applied topical CHM as a heat pack, using the topical CHM formula *Xiao tong san* 消痛散, which contained three herbs: *Tu si zi* 菟丝子, *lai fu zi* 莱菔子 and *bu gu zhi* 补骨脂. As orally used CHM, one commercialised CHM product, *Jing tong* granule 颈痛颗粒, was assessed by four RCTs (C5, C6, C13, C15). The other four RCTs (C3, C8, C10, C11) used self-prescribed oral CHM formulae in a decoction form, but did not provide the formula names. Among the seven RCTs that used oral CHM formulae, the most common CHM herbs were: *Bai shao* 白芍 (*n* = 8), *ge gen* 葛根 (*n* = 7), *chuan xiong* 川芎 (*n* = 6), *san qi* 三七) (*n* = 5), *wei ling tian* 威灵仙 (*n* = 5), *yan hu suo* 延胡索 (*n* = 5) and *qiang huo* 羌活 (*n* = 5).

Twelve RCTs (C1, C2, C4, C7–C12, C16–C18) reported information on acupuncture points; one RCT (C11) used these points for *tuina* 推拿 therapy: GB20 *Fengchi* 风池, LI18 *Futu* 扶突, GV16 *Fengfu* 风府, GB21 *Jiangjin* 肩井, and SI11 *Tianzong* 天宗. The other 11 RCTs applied acupuncture therapy on varied points; the common ones were: Cervical EX-B2 *Jiaji* 颈夹脊 points (*n* = 8),

GB20 *Fengchi* 风池 (*n* = 8), GB21 *Jiangjin* 肩井 (*n* = 7), LI11 *Quchi* 曲池 (*n* = 5), LI4 *Hegu* 合谷 (*n* = 4), SI3 *Houxi* 后溪 (*n* = 4), TE5 *Waiguan* 外关 (*n* = 4), SI11 *Tianzong* 天宗 (*n* = 4) and GV14 *Dazhui* 大椎 (*n* = 3).

The treatment effects of Chinese medicine combination therapy are presented in line with the types of treatment and control intervention. Since Chinese medicine therapies and routine care therapies varied across studies, meta-analysis was not feasible for most comparisons.

Risk-of-Bias Assessment

All included studies were described as RCTs. However, only ten studies stated an appropriate method for randomisation sequence generation, and therefore they were assessed as "low" risk of bias for this domain; the remaining studies were of "unclear" risk due to a lack of information. For allocation concealment, two studies that centred randomisation properly concealed the group allocation, and two studies used the opaque envelope method; they were assessed as "low" risk of bias. The other studies were of "unclear" risk due to a lack of information. All studies were assessed as "high" risk for blinding (of participants, personnel and outcome assessors) because they applied different therapies in the intervention and control groups and did not make any effort to achieve blinding.

Incomplete outcome data was assessed to be of "low" risk of bias for 16 studies since there were no dropouts in these studies. Two studies were at "unclear" risk for this because it was not clear whether there were dropouts. One study was assessed as an "high" risk for selective reporting because it did not report all outcomes defined in its methods section; the other studies were also assessed as "unclear" risks since their protocols could not be identified. See Table 9.2 for a summary.

The effects of Chinese medicine combination therapy are presented under each category of combination therapy as following.

Table 9.2.   Risk-of-Bias Assessment of Randomised Controlled Trials

Risk-of-Bias Domain	Low Risk *n* (%)	Unclear Risk *n* (%)	High Risk *n* (%)
Sequence generation	10 (55.6)	8 (44.4)	0 (0)
Allocation concealment	4 (22.2)	14 (77.8)	0 (0)
Blinding of participants	0 (0)	0 (0)	18 (100)
Blinding of personnel*	0 (0)	0 (0)	18 (100)
Blinding of outcome assessors	0 (0)	0 (0)	18 (100)
Incomplete outcome data	16 (88.9)	2 (11.1)	0 (0)
Selective outcome reporting	0 (0)	17 (94.4)	1 (5.6)

*Blinding of personnel is challenging in manual therapies.

Chinese Herbal Medicine and Acupuncture

Two RCTs (C8, C10) evaluated a combination of CHM and acupuncture. Yang's study (C8) in 2016 compared the combination of the oral CHM *Ge gen tang* 葛根汤 and acupuncture with pharmacotherapy (ibuprofen), using the effective rate and pain Visual Analogue Scale (VAS) as the outcome measure; 82 participants were involved in this study. After two weeks of treatment, participants in the Chinese medicine group achieved better effects in terms of the effective rate and pain VAS than those who received ibuprofen.

Wang's study (C10) in 2005 assessed the add-on effect of CHM and acupuncture to pharmacotherapy plus traction therapy. This study specifically recruited 123 patients aged between 50 and 75 years old who had the Chinese medicine syndrome of *yang* deficiency and coldness stagnation 虚寒型. Participants received acupuncture and the oral CHM *Huang qi gui zhi wu wu tang* 黄芪桂枝五物汤 in addition to pharmacotherapy plus traction therapy compared to just pharmacotherapy plus traction therapy. This study used the effective rate and the Scoring System for Cervical Radiculopathy (SSCR) as the outcome measures. Superior effects were reported in the Chinese medicine group for both outcome measures at the end of the treatment phase and after a three-month follow-up phase.

Chinese Herbal Medicine and *Tuina* 推拿 Therapy

Three studies (C3, C11, C14) evaluated the treatment effects of CHM in combination with *tuina* 推拿 therapy, using routine care therapies as the comparators.

Zhang's study (C3) in 2018 compared a combination of CHM and *tuina* 推拿 therapy with pharmacotherapy (celecoxib capsules and mecobalamin). Oral CHM was prescribed according to the participants' Chinese medicine syndrome types. *Tuina* 推拿 therapy was administered once daily. A total of 60 participants was included in this study. All participants received two weeks of treatment. The study reported that the Chinese medicine treatments were more effective than the control for both the VAS and Neck Disability Index (NDI) at the end of the treatment phase and the follow-up phase (12 weeks after treatment had ended).

Tang's study (C11) in 2013 compared a combination of oral CHM and *tuina* 推拿 therapy with traction therapy plus pharmacotherapy (celecoxib capsules). In this study, the oral CHM *Ge gen tang* 葛根汤 was prescribed, allowing individualised modification according to the participants' syndrome differentiation. *Tuina* 推拿 therapy was administered once every two days. Traction therapy was applied once daily. All participants received two weeks of treatment. The Chinese medicine group achieved better treatment effects than the routine care group in terms of the pain VAS and effective rate.

Zhang's study (C14) in 2010 compared a combination of topical CHM and *tuina* 推拿 therapy with traction therapy. A total of 100 participants with wind-cold blocking meridians 风寒阻络 syndrome was included in this study. The topical CHM *Xiao tong san* 消痛散 was applied as a heat pack in the neck region. All therapies were administered once a day, continually for two weeks. Chinese medicine therapies were more effective than traction therapy in terms of the effective rate and pain VAS.

All these three studies reported data on the VAS. Meta-analysis results showed that the overall effect of CHM in combination with *tuina* 推拿 therapy was superior to routine care therapies (3 studies, MD: −1.13 [−1.49, −0.76], I^2 = 0%). However, since the CHM therapy was used either orally or topically, and the routine care therapies varied in these three studies, the meta-analysis result should be interpreted with caution.

Chinese Herbal Medicine and *Tuina* 推拿 Therapy and *Daoyin* 导引 Exercise

Four studies (C5, C6, C13, C15) evaluated the effects of CHM plus *tuina* 推拿 therapy and *daoyin* 导引 exercise. Three studies (C5, C6, C13) compared the Chinese medicine combination therapy with routine care therapies (pharmacotherapy plus traction therapy); all three reported data on the effective rate. The meta-analysis result showed that there was no significant difference between the Chinese medicine combination therapy and routine care therapies (RR: 1.56 [1.00, 2.42], I^2 = 97%). It is worth noting that all three studies reported follow-up data; Liu's study (C5) in 2013 reported the recurrence rate at one month after the treatment phase, while his 2016 study (C6) reported this at five years after the treatment phase. Zhen's study (C13) in 2010 reported the cervical range of motion at the end of a six-month follow-up phase. All three studies concluded that Chinese medicine therapies had a better long-term effect than routine care therapies.

One study (C15) evaluated the add-on effect of CHM plus *tuina* 推拿 therapy and *daoyin* 导引 exercise to a combination of diclofenac tablets plus traction therapy. After two weeks, Chinese medicine therapies were found to have significant add-on effects in terms of the effective rate and symptoms scores.

Acupuncture and *Tuina* 推拿 Therapy

The combination of acupuncture and *tuina* 推拿 therapy was evaluated in four studies (C4, C7, C9, C18). Two studies (C4, C18) applied electroacupuncture, and the other two (C7, C9) used a normal acupuncture needling method.

All four studies reported data on the effective rate. and the meta-analysis result showed that the combination of acupuncture and *tuina* 推拿 therapy was more effective than routine care therapies

(4 Studies, RR: 1.13 [1.04, 1.23], I^2 = 20%). However, the intervention and control therapies used in these four studies varied. Details of each study are described below.

Two studies evaluated electroacupuncture in combination with *tuina* 推拿 therapy. Zhang's study (C4) in 2015 compared a Chinese medicine combination therapy with diclofenac tablets plus traction therapy for 20 days; the Chinese medicine combination therapy was more effective than routine care therapies for the effective rate and pain VAS. Zeng's study (C18) in 2014 compared a combination with traction therapy. Electroacupuncture, *tuina* 推拿 therapy and traction therapy were administered three times a week for a total duration of four weeks. A post-treatment between-group comparison showed that the Chinese medicine combination therapy was more effective for the effective rate, McGill Pain Questionnaire (MPQ), NDI and SSCR scores.

Two studies (C7, C9) used acupuncture and *tuina* 推拿 as the Chinese medicine combination therapy. One study (C7) compared this combination to traction therapy plus physiotherapy using a low-frequency electric therapy apparatus. All treatments were applied once a day, for a total of 21 days. This study reported data only on the effective rate, with the result favouring the Chinese medicine combination therapy. The other study (C9) compared a combination of acupuncture and *tuina* 推拿 therapy with traction therapy. All these therapies were administered once every two days. After two weeks of treatment, the Chinese medicine combination therapy achieved better effects in terms of the effective rate and the Outcome Assessment System in the Treatment of Cervical Radiculopathy (OASTCR) score.

Electroacupuncture and Cupping

Two studies (C12, C16) evaluated the effect of electroacupuncture plus cupping. One study (C12) compared a combination of electroacupuncture and cupping with traction therapy for 20 days, reporting that the Chinese medicine combination therapy was more effective in terms of the effective rate and MPQ. The other study (C16) compared the combination with meloxicam tablets for 20 days, showing that there was no significant difference between the Chinese medicine therapies and meloxicam for the effective rate.

Both studies reported data on the effective rate, and the meta-analysis result showed that the combination of electroacupuncture plus cupping was not significantly different to routine care therapies (2 studies, RR: 1.20 [0.60, 2.39], I^2 = 90%).

Acupuncture and *Daoyin* 导引 Exercise

One study (C1) evaluated the add-on effect of acupuncture and *daoyin* 导引 exercise to a combination of traction therapy and diclofenac tablets. The effective rate, pain VAS and Clinical Assessment Scale for Cervical Spondylosis (CASCS) were used as outcome measures. After 15 days of treatment, the Chinese medicine combination therapy achieved better effects for all three outcome measures.

Acupuncture and *Tuina* 推拿 Therapy and *Daoyin* 导引 Exercise

Two studies (C2, C17) applied a combination of acupuncture plus *tuina* 推拿 therapy and *daoyin* 导引 exercise as an add-on therapy to a combination of traction therapy and physiotherapy using an infrared lamp. A total of 726 participants were included in these two studies. Both studies reported data on the effective rate and meta-analysis showed there was no significant difference between the Chinese medicine combination therapy and the routine care (2 studies, RR: 1.00 [0.97, 1.03], I^2 = 0%).

Assessment Using Grading of Recommendations Assessment, Development and Evaluation

Using the Grading of Recommendations Assessment, Development and Evaluation (GRADE) approach, the certainty of evidence for the combination of acupuncture and *tuina* 推拿 therapy was assessed as

Table 9.3.   GRADE: Acupuncture Plus *Tuina* 推拿 Therapy *vs*. Routine Care

Outcome (End of Treatment)	Absolute Effect		Relative Effect (95% CI) No. of Participants (Studies)	Certainty of Evidence (GRADE)
	Acupuncture plus *Tuina* (推拿) Therapy	Routine Care		
Effective rate	**86** per 100	76 per 100	**RR 1.13** (1.04, 1.23)	⊕⊕○○ LOW[1,2]
	Difference: 10 more per 100 patients (95% CI: 3 more to 18 more per 100 patients)		416 (4 RCTs)	

The risk in the intervention group (and its 95% CI) is based on the assumed risk in the comparison group and the relative effect of the intervention (and its 95% CI).

Abbreviations: CI, confidence interval; GRADE, Grading of Recommendations Assessment, Development and Evaluation; RCT, randomised controlled trial; RR, risk ratio.

Notes:
1) Lack of blinding of participants and personnel may have influenced results;
2) Small sample sizes may have limited the certainty of results; and
3) High heterogeneity may have limited the certainty of results.

Study reference:
Effective rate: C4, C7, C9, C18

"low". The small sample size and the lack of blinding in the design of RCTs downgraded the certainty of the evidence (Table 9.3).

Non-Controlled Studies

A total of 37 case series studies (C19–C47, C49–C56) and one case report (C48) were identified through our comprehensive search, with a total of 2,880 patients being involved in these studies.

All these studies applied more than one type of Chinese medicine therapies and the combinations were:

- CHM and acupuncture therapies: Four studies (C29, C39, C54, C56);
- CHM and *tuina* 推拿 therapy: 16 studies (C20, C26, C27, C30, C31, C35, C37, C41–C43, C45–C47, C49, C50, C55);

- CHM and acupuncture and *tuina* 推拿 therapy: Four studies (C19, C25, C36, C44);
- Acupuncture and *tuina* 推拿 therapy: 13 studies (C21–C24, C32–C34, C38, C40, C48, C51–C53); and
- CHM and *daoyin* 导引 exercise: One study (C28).

The Chinese medicine syndrome differentiation approach was applied in two studies (C36, C39) to prescribe treatments accordingly. The syndromes mentioned in these two studies were: wind-cold blocking meridians 风寒痹阻, *qi* stagnation and Blood stasis 气滞血瘀 and Liver-Spleen-Kidney deficiency 肝脾肾亏虚.

The CHM formulas investigated by these studies varied. One CHM commercial product, *Jing tong* granule 颈痛颗粒, was evaluated by multiple studies (C41, C42, C44, C47). All CHM formulae contained multiple herb ingredients. The most commonly used herbs were: *Bai shao* 白芍 ($n = 20$), *chuan xiong* 川芎 ($n = 22$), *ge gen* 葛根 ($n = 20$), *dang gui* 当归 ($n = 16$), *qiang huo* 羌活 ($n = 15$), *wei ling xian* 威灵仙 ($n = 13$), *gui zhi* 桂枝 ($n = 13$), *ji xue teng* 鸡血藤 ($n = 12$), *di huang* 地黄 ($n = 12$) and *huang qi* 黄芪 ($n = 9$).

In terms of the points used for acupuncture and other types of Chinese medicine therapies, the commonly used ones were: GB20 *Fengchi* 风池 ($n = 18$), GB21 *Jianjing* 肩井 ($n = 17$), LI11 *Quchi* 曲池 ($n = 14$), cervical EX-B2 *Jiaji* 颈夹脊 points ($n = 13$), LI4 *Hegu* 合谷 ($n = 11$), GV14 *Dazhui* 大椎 ($n = 11$), *Ashi* points 阿是穴 ($n = 10$), SI3 *Houzi* 后溪 ($n = 9$), TE5 *Waiguan* 外关 ($n = 9$), TE11 *Tianzong* 天宗 ($n = 9$), TE15 *Jianzhongshu* 肩中俞 ($n = 9$) and GV16 *Fengfu* 风府 ($n = 9$).

Safety of Chinese Medicine Combination Therapy

Safety information on the Chinese medicine therapies was reported in two RCTs (C8, C10) and one non-controlled study (C46). In these three studies, among a total of 149 participants who received CHM treatment, nine occasions of mild gastrointestinal symptoms after taking CHM were recorded. All these episodes resolved themselves without any additional management required. Other included studies did not report information related to adverse events (AEs).

Evidence for Chinese Medicine Combination Therapy Commonly Used in Clinical Practice

In the clinical research on Chinese medicine combination therapy, two or more different types of Chinese medicine therapies were combined: CHM, acupuncture, *tuina* 推拿 therapy, cupping and *daoyin* 导引 exercise. This could be interpreted as it being common to combine two or more Chinese medicine therapies in the management of CR in clinical practice. All of these therapies were recommended in Chapter 2, although there were no specific recommendations on which should be combined (see Chapter 2).

The CHM formulae and herbs, acupuncture methods and points, and *tuina* 推拿 therapy methods used in the combination therapy were consistent with those recommended in Chapter 2 and those evaluated as single treatments (see Chapters 5, 7 and 8).

Summary of Chinese Medicine Combination Therapy Clinical Evidence

There is some clinical research evidence showing the results of Chinese medicine combination therapy as treatments for CR. Since the therapies used in the included studies varied, meta-analysis was not feasible for every type of combination. Our evaluation showed that:

- CHM plus *tuina* 推拿 therapy was more effective than routine care therapies for the pain VAS (meta-analysis of three RCTs);
- CHM plus *tuina* 推拿 therapy and *daoyin* 导引 exercise was no different to routine care therapies for the effective rate (meta-analysis of four RCTs);
- Acupuncture plus *tuina* 推拿 therapy was more effective than routine care therapies for the effective rate (meta-analysis of four RCTs);

- Electroacupuncture plus cupping was no different to routine care therapies for the effective rate (meta-analysis of two RCTs); and
- Acupuncture plus *tuina* 推拿 therapy and *daoyin* 导引 exercise was not a significantly effective add-on therapy to routine care therapies for the effective rate (meta-analysis of two RCTs).

It is interesting to note that combining two or three different types of Chinese medicine therapies does not seem to be more effective than applying one type of Chinese medicine therapy in the treatment of CR. However, since we did not include studies comparing only different Chinese medicine therapies, such a trend could not be confirmed.

The commonly used CHM formulae and herbs, acupuncture points and methods, and details of other Chinese medicine therapies are consistent with those summarised in Chapters 5, 7 and 8. The common treatment duration was two weeks to 20 days. Except for mild gastrointestinal symptoms related to CHM, there were no other AEs reported.

References

1. 中华中医药学会. (2008) 中医内科常见病诊疗指南—西医疾病部分. 中国中医药出版社, 北京, 143–147.
2. 屈松柏, 李家庚. (2000) 实用中医心血管病学. 第 2 版. 科学技术文献出版社, 北京.

References to Included Clinical Studies

Study ID	Reference
C1	朱艳风, 刘士诚, 韩昆, *et al.* (2017) 针刺运动疗法结合益颈通络经对青年颈椎病患者颈椎曲度的影响. *现代中西医结合杂志* **26**(25): 2779–2781.
C2	周建伟, 蒋振亚, 叶锐彬, *et al.* (2006) 针灸推拿为主治疗神经根型颈椎病: 多中心随机对照研究. *中国针灸* **26**(8): 537–543.

(*Continued*)

Study ID	Reference
C3	张洋, 程少丹, 葛程, *et al.* (2018) 整颈三步九法结合中药治疗神经根型颈椎病的临床研究. *中国中医骨伤科杂志* **26**(6): 34–37.
C4	张少林, 王明, 王平, 穆刚. (2015) 推拿手法配合电针治疗神经根型颈椎病临床研究. *陕西中医* **36**(8): 1059–1060.
C5	于杰, 朱立国, 李俊杰, *et al.* (2013) 中医综合疗法治疗神经根型颈椎病后肩臂疼痛症状复发率的临床研究. *北京中医药* **32**(12): 885–888.
C6	于杰, 朱立国, 洪毅, *et al.* (2016) 中医综合疗法治疗神经根型颈椎病的疗效评价与长期随访. *中国中医骨伤科杂志* **24**: 11–13, 17.
C7	尹利华, 张细銮, 谢建平, *et al.* (2009) 针刺配合手法治疗神经根型颈椎病 60 例. *江西中医药* **40**(8): 65–66.
C8	杨茜, 彭新. (2016) 针灸联合桂枝加葛根汤治疗神经根型颈椎病临床疗效观察. *针灸临床杂志* **32**(10): 29–31.
C9	吴江林, 林定坤, 陈博来, *et al.* (2012) 手法配合颈痛穴针刺治疗神经根型颈椎病临床观察. *新中医* **44**(5): 107–109.
C10	王羽丰, 邓晋丰, 林定坤, *et al.* (2005) 中医综合疗法治疗老年虚寒型神经根型颈椎病的临床研究. *中国中医骨伤科杂志* **13**(6): 21–24.
C11	唐汉武, 孙丽, 黄承军. (2013) 手法配合中药内服治疗神经根型颈椎病的临床观察. *颈腰痛杂志* **34**(2): 173–175.
C12	李婕, 谢玮, 范伟强, *et al.* (2018) "颈七针"治疗神经根型颈椎病疗效观察. *上海针灸杂志* **37**(2): 222–225.
C13	甄朋超. (2010) 中医综合疗法对神经根型颈椎病颈椎 ROM 改善的临床研究 (Thesis). 中国中医科学院.
C14	张旭东. (2010) 颈项牵旋法结合消痛散外熨法治疗神经根型颈椎病的临床研究 (Thesis). 长春中医药大学.
C15	吴江林. (2009) 中医综合疗法治疗神经根型颈椎病疗效和安全性研究 (Thesis). 广州中医药大学.
C16	刘素君, 梁晶, 潘超安, *et al.* (2016) 针罐结合治疗神经根型颈椎病的临床疗效观察(英文). *J Acupunct Tuina Sci* **14**(04): 290–294.
C17	李德华. (2006) 五联综合疗法治疗颈椎病（神经根型）的临床研究 (Thesis). 成都中医药大学.
C18	曾景钊. (2014) 电针结合推拿治疗神经根型颈椎病的临床疗效观察 (Thesis). 广州中医药大学.
C19	朱志峰. (2017) 澄江针伤五步法治疗神经根型颈椎病60例. *河南中医* **37**(12): 2205–2207.

(*Continued*)

(*Continued*)

Study ID	Reference
C20	朱立国, 高景华, 李金学, *et al.* (2011) 项痹病(神经根型颈椎病)诊疗方案验证. *北京中医药* **30**(4): 254–257.
C21	张志松. (2007) 定点旋扳配合电针治疗神经根型颈椎病 180 例. *针灸临床杂志* **23**(5): 13.
C22	张永泉, 王平. (2011) 先旋再提手法结合针刺治疗神经根型颈椎病 31 例. *中国中医急症* **20**(11): 1875.
C23	张梦佛. (2012) 推拿手法结合针刺后溪治疗神经根型颈椎病 31 例. *按摩与康复医学* **3**(36): 85.
C24	张凯. (2011) 针刺及推拿治疗神经根型颈椎病 50 例. *中国中医急症* **20**(6): 989–990.
C25	张殿银, 刘菲菲. (2016) 海桐皮汤热敷配合针灸推拿治疗神经根型颈椎病的临床观察. *山西医药杂志* **45**(18): 2192–2193.
C26	于向荣, 姚敏. (2011) 中药内服配合推拿手法治疗神经根型颈椎病 82 例. *现代中医药* **31**(1): 35.
C27	游力. (2010) 37 例神经根型颈椎病中药治疗效果分析. *中国中医药咨讯* **2**(1): 102–103.
C28	叶秀兰, 王拥军. (2001) 中药结合操练治疗神经根型颈椎病 72 例报告. *中医正骨* **13**(6): 25–26.
C29	叶梅惠. (2017) 针药结合治疗神经根型颈椎病 65 例疗效观察. *云南中医中药杂志* **38**(11): 64–65.
C30	杨桦, 王虹. (2005) 推拿手法配合芍药加味汤治疗神经根型颈椎病 40 例. *陕西中医* **26**(4): 330–331.
C31	杨昌金. (2009) 推拿结合中药内服治疗神经根型颈椎病 50 例. *黑龙江中医药* (4): 32–33.
C32	杨爱国. (2013) 针刺配合手法治疗神经根型颈椎病 80 例. *广西中医药大学学报* **16**(2): 534.
C33	薛传疆, 方志远. (2014) 手法加针刺治疗神经根型颈椎病 45 例. *国际中医中药杂志* **36**(6): 563.
C34	吴新忠. (2009) 输短刺配合手法治疗神经根型颈椎病的疗效观察. *当代医学* **15**(33): 156.
C35	吴国成, 王得斌. (2009) 手法配合中药熏洗热敷治疗神经根型颈椎病 54 例. *甘肃中医* **22**(5): 28–29.
C36	魏林, 赵海华, 刘卫. (2016) 辨证分型治疗神经根型颈椎病 118 例观察. *中医临床研究* **8**(22): 86–87.

(*Continued*)

Study ID	Reference
C37	王少伟, 郑志辉. (2012) 动点定位旋扳手法配合中药治疗神经根型颈椎病疗效观察. *新中医* **44**(7): 132–134.
C38	万金来, 杜跃. (2006) 针灸配合定位旋转复位法治疗神经根型颈椎病 78 例疗效观察. *河北中医药学报* **21**(2): 31–32.
C39	田江波, 张赛冲. (2012) 电针配合口服中药治疗神经根型颈椎病 60 例临床观察. *中国实用医药* **7**(11): 145–146.
C40	唐流刚, 喻杉, 吴晓惠, 王标. (2015) 经斜角肌间沟电针手法治疗神经根型颈椎病 100 例疗效观察. *四川中医* **33**(9): 158–159.
C41	石震, 闫素敏, 戈超, 陈锋. (2014) 整脊疗法配合颈痛颗粒治疗神经根型颈椎病 150 例. *实用中医药杂志* **30**(3): 194.
C42	马善治, 郭剑华, 刘渝松, *et al.* (2010) 神经根型颈椎病诊疗方案临床验证报告. *实用中医药杂志* **26**(2): 85–86.
C43	刘玉峰, 王平, 李远栋. (2012) 小角度提拉手法配合中药治疗神经根型颈椎病 37 例. *江西中医药* **43**(8): 46–48.
C44	李洲进, 吴官保, 汤伟. (2011) 颈痛颗粒配合针灸推拿治疗神经根型颈椎病 65 例临床观察. *中国中医药咨讯* **3**(5): 49.
C45	郭小伟, 张建福. (2013) 宣痹舒络汤配合提牵旋转手法治疗神经根型颈椎病临床观察. *中医学报* **28**(12): 1918–1919.
C46	顾家龙. (2013) 自拟葛芍威舒痹汤配合旋提手法治疗神经根型颈椎病 42 例. *广西中医药大学学报* **16**(2): 55–56.
C47	陈欣, 席芳琴, 郭铁峰, 顾玉彪. (2010) 三步理筋手法联合颈痛颗粒治疗神经根型颈椎病 30 例. *中国中医骨伤科杂志* **18**(7): 23–24.
C48	陈涛, 时圣瑞, 左海峰, 王遵来. (2018) 三小定点整脊手法联合针刺治疗神经根型颈椎病. *吉林中医药* **38**(4): 448–451.
C49	张志文, 冯卫星, 张扬立, 李福林. (2008) 中药配合推拿治疗神经根型颈椎病 36 例. *甘肃中医* **21**(8): 34–35.
C50	赵立平, 罗光文, 李志峰. (2004) 推拿配合桂枝加葛根汤治疗神经根型颈椎病 60 例. *河北中医* **26**(11): 849.
C51	袁国华, 刘秋菊, 张鹏. (2014) 温针结合推拿治疗颈椎病 62 例. *中医外治杂志* **23**(5): 44–45.
C52	杨彬, 史晓菲. (2012) 手法配合针灸治疗神经根型颈椎病 80 例临床观察. *中外健康文摘* **30**(3): 253–254.
C53	韦莉莉. (2005) 电针配合手法治疗神经根型颈椎病 88 例. *浙江中医学院学报* **29**(2): 68.

(*Continued*)

Study ID	Reference
C54	罗琳. (2013) 针刺配合中药湿热敷治疗神经根型颈椎病 118 例. *云南中医中药杂志* **34**(11): 57–58.
C55	刘青, 詹先蓉, 周菊芳. (2000) 中药内服配合推拿治疗神经根型颈椎病 50 例. *四川中医* **18**(7): 49–50.
C56	李鸿霞. (2011) 针刺药灸配合耳穴治疗神经根型颈椎病 35 例. *中医药导报* **17**(12): 61–62.

10

Summary of Evidence

OVERVIEW

Chinese medicine therapies have been used to treat cervical radiculopathy for a long time. In recent decades, a number of clinical studies have been conducted to evaluate Chinese medicine therapies. Findings from clinical evidence revealed promising benefits of Chinese herbal medicine, acupuncture and other Chinese medicine therapies. This chapter provides a "whole evidence" analysis of Chinese medicine for the management of cervical radiculopathy. The limitations of the available evidence are discussed and future directions are identified for further clinical and experimental research.

Introduction

Cervical radiculopathy (CR) is defined as *"pain in a radicular pattern in one or both upper extremities related to compression and/ or irritation of one or more cervical nerve roots. Frequent signs and symptoms include varying degrees of sensory, motor, and reflex changes as well as dysesthesias and paresthesias related to nerve roots without evidence of spinal cord dysfunction (myelopathy)"*.[1] Typical symptoms of CR include neck pain, unilateral or bilateral radiating arm pain, paraesthesia, sensory or motor deficits, and reflex impairment or loss in the upper extremities and neck. These symptoms usually present in a dermatome pattern according to the different levels of compression of nerve roots.[2,3] Cervical radiculopathy occurs in people of any age group, with those aged around 50 years being the most common group.[3,4] The main symptom of

CR, neck pain, has been found to be associated with a high economic burden. Cervical disc degeneration and cervical spondylosis pathologies have been identified as the main pathological causes of CR.[5–7]

In clinical management, the preliminary goal of CR management is to minimise pain, improve neurological function and prevent recurrence.[2,7] Pharmacotherapies, surgical interventions and physiotherapy are recommended by current clinical guidelines for CR management.[1,5,8]

Chinese medicine therapies have played a long-term role in the management of CR. In order to provide a "whole evidence" evaluation, we analysed the evidence on Chinese medicine therapies for CR from all types of literature in this monograph.

A review of clinical guidelines and textbooks identified a range of Chinese medicine treatments that have been recommended or suggested, including oral or topical Chinese herbal medicine (CHM), acupuncture-related therapies, cupping, *tuina* 推拿 therapy and *daoyin* 导引 exercise (Chapter 2).

Considering that CR was not systematically discussed in history, identifying effective Chinese medicine treatments from classical literature is challenging. This condition was likely considered a part of *Bi* disease 痹证. In addition, the relevant symptoms of CR are recorded in classical literature under various terms that describe its symptoms or anatomical locations. Therefore, we conducted a comprehensive search in the digital collections of the Chinese medicine book *Zhong Hua Yi Dian* 中华医典 to locate relevant treatments used in history (Chapter 3).

Many clinical trials of Chinese medicine therapies have been conducted in China. Some of these studies have shown promising results. Using a systematic review approach (Chapter 4), clinical evidence was found to support the use of oral CHM (Chapter 5), acupuncture therapies (Chapter 7), *tuina* 推拿 therapy (Chapter 8) and some combinations of multiple Chinese medicine therapies (Chapter 9). The herbs that were used most frequently in clinical studies have shown actions in experimental studies that shed light on their probable mechanisms of action (Chapter 6).

Chinese Medicine Syndrome Differentiation

As summarised in Chapter 2, the Chinese medicine aetiology and pathogenesis of CR introduced in current clinical guidelines are a combination of a weak constitution, muscle strain or injury, and invasion of external pathogens. Clinically, patients may present one or more of the following syndromes: Wind-cold blocking meridians 风寒痹阻, *qi* stagnation and Blood stasis 气滞血瘀, phlegm and dampness blocking meridians 痰湿阻络, Liver and Kidney deficiency 肝肾不足, and *qi* and Blood deficiency 气血亏虚.

The aetiology of CR recorded in classical literature was grouped into external factors (wind, cold and dampness) and internal factors (*qi* and Blood deficiency 气血亏虚, lack of nourishment for meridians 经脉失养 and internal phlegm 痰饮, as well as traumatic injury).

In clinical studies, information on Chinese medicine syndrome differentiation was often not reported (see Chapters 5, 7, 8 and 9). Based on the information collected from some of the clinical studies included in our evaluations, the common Chinese medicine syndrome differentiation types were *qi* stagnation and Blood stasis 气滞血瘀 and wind-cold-dampness invasion 风寒湿证.

Comparing the main syndromes introduced in Chapters 2, 3 and 5, it could clearly be seen that the key syndromes of CR were consistent across all types of evidence. Clinical management should consider relieving symptoms in line with addressing the Chinese medicine syndromes, in particular, using oral CHM treatments. However, although some clinical studies used syndrome differentiation for treatment selection (especially when multiple formulae were used in one study), results were usually reported in aggregate and not by syndrome type. Hence, it was not possible to conduct subgroup analyses based on the syndrome type to establish the efficacy of treatments according to specific syndrome types.

Chinese Herbal Medicine

This section summarises the evidence from Chapters 2, 3, 5 and 9.

CHM therapies have been documented in all forms as evidence for managing CR. Oral CHM is recommended to be applied according to the Chinese medicine syndrome and clinicians may select corresponding CHM formulae or herbs when syndrome differentiation diagnosis is determined. Focusing on the main syndrome types for CR listed by the contemporary literature, the following formulas can be considered and may be used with modifications or in combination based on individual syndrome differentiation: *Qiang huo sheng shi tang* 羌活胜湿汤, *Shu feng huo xue tang* 疏风活血汤, *Juan bi tang* 蠲痹汤, *Tao hong si wu tang* 桃红四物汤, *Shen tong zhu yu tang* 身痛逐瘀汤, *Ban xia bai zhu tian ma tang* 半夏白术天麻汤, *Shen qi wan* 肾气丸, *Du huo ji sheng tang* 独活寄生汤, *Huang qi gui zhi wu wu tang* 黄芪桂枝五物汤, and *Ba zhen tang* 八珍汤 (see Chapter 2 for more details). CHM is also recommended to be applied externally.

In the evaluation of modern literature evidence on CHM for CR (Chapter 5), it was found that both oral CHM and topical CHM treatments provided some evidence in clinical research. In terms of oral CHM formulae, our evaluation of clinical studies identified no classical CHM formulae used in multiple randomised controlled trials (RCTs) and one oral CHM formula *Huang qi gui zhi wu wu tang* 黄芪桂枝五物汤 reported in three non-controlled clinical studies. Although there was no high-level uniformity in terms of the CHM formula names, there were similarities in the herbs used in the included studies. The most commonly used herbs were: *Ge gen* 葛根, *bai shao* 白芍/chi shao 赤芍, *huang qi* 黄芪, *gui zhi* 桂枝, *chuan xiong* 川芎, *dang gui* 当归, *gan cao* 甘草 and *qiang huo* 羌活. In the RCTs evaluated, an externally applied CHM therapy also used similar herbs. When CHM was used externally, they were made as CHM ointments, CHM heat packs or CHM decoctions applied using a device that assisted the process of transdermal drug delivery.

By reviewing the available experimental evidence, it was found that the most frequently used Chinese herbs were associated with some possible biological activities and mechanisms relevant to CR (Chapter 6). In particular, one commercialised oral CHM product, *Gen tong ping ke li* 根痛平颗粒, was shown to improve motor function recovery and decrease neuropathic pain. From a Chinese medicine perspective, this product functions by promoting *qi* to activate Blood and by removing meridian obstruction to relieve pain (行气活血, 通络止痛). This formula also has been proven effective for improving motor function recovery and somatosensory-evoked potentials by pre-clinical research (see Chapter 6).

The clinical research showed that oral CHM was more effective than routine care therapies; oral CHM plus routine care therapies were more effective than routine care therapies alone, and topical CHM was more effective than routine care therapies. All these superior effects were found in multiple outcome measures. However, the certainty of most of the evidence was "low" as shown by the Grading of Recommendations Assessment, Development and Evaluation (GRADE) assessment (see Chapter 5 for more details).

In order to provide evidence regarding the possible effective herbs used in clinical practice, the most frequent herbs used in the studies were calculated from favourable meta-analyses. Studies were pooled according to six main outcome measure groups regardless of their comparator: (1) Effective rate, (2) Pain, and (3) CR-specific outcomes. The herbs used in the RCTs and included in positive meta-analyses were similar across different types of outcomes and also consistent with the overall most common herbs. It could be concluded that the herbs *shao yao* 芍药 (including *bai shao* 白芍, *chi shao* 赤芍 or *shao yao* 芍药), *ge gen* 葛根, *gan cao* 甘草, *chuan xiong* 川芎, *fu zi* 附子/*wu tou* 乌头 and *gui zhi* 桂枝 may be effective for the management of CR in oral CHM, while *fu zi* 附子/*wu tou* 乌头, *wei ling xian* 威灵仙, *dang gui* 当归 and *hong hua* 红花 may be the effective herbs for topical application. *Fu zi* 附子/*wu tou* 乌头 is considered effective for pain relief but may be restricted in some countries, and readers are advised to pay attention to the toxicity of these herbs and to comply with relevant regulations.

Adverse events (AEs) related to CHM were rarely reported, indicating that CHM may be safe. However, most of the included studies did not mention information on AEs, and therefore poor reporting may have caused safety issues in relation to CHM not being fully disclosed.

The heterogeneity in the meta-analyses indicates that there was considerable variability in each result. At least part of this variability was due to the use of different CHMs, but it was not possible for us to determine which CHM produced the greatest effects, since most studies tested different formulae, even when they were based on similar ingredients. Other factors influencing the interpretation of the results of the clinical studies were the diversity of treatment duration and disease severity. Since the numbers of studies included in each meta-analysis were quite small, subgroup meta-analyses were not feasible in most cases. These aspects have reduced confidence in the accuracy of the reported results and influenced the downgrading of the certainty of the evidence in the GRADE assessments.

Chinese Herbal Medicine Formulae in Key Clinical Guidelines and Textbooks, Classical Literature and Clinical Studies

Table 10.1 summarises the oral CHM formulae described in the clinical guidelines and textbooks (Chapter 2), classical literature (Chapter 3) and clinical studies (Chapter 5). Assessment was based on formula name. It is likely that formulae with the same or similar herb ingredients, but different formula names were also included in the classical literature and clinical research. Since assessment of the similarity of formulae is complex and was not undertaken, the actual number of occurrences of each listed formula may be higher than reported (Table 10.1).

The formulae recorded in classical literature were not fully incon-sistent with those commonly used in current clinical practice. *Qiang huo sheng shi tang* 羌活胜湿汤 is the only CHM formula that pro-vided evidence from all categories of evidence: Contemporary literature (Chapter 2), classical literature (Chapter 3) and clinical studies (Chapter 9); *Juan bi tang* 蠲痹汤 is recommended by clinical guidelines or textbooks as well as being recorded in classical litera-ture, and *Shen tong zhu yu tang* 身痛逐瘀汤 and *Huang qi gui zhi wu wu tang* 黄芪桂枝五物汤 are recommended by contemporary

Table 10.1. Summary of Oral Chinese Herbal Medicine Formulae

Formula Name	Evidence in Clinical Guidelines and Textbooks (Chapter 2)	Evidence in Classical Literature (Chapter 3) (No. of Citations)	Included in Clinical Studies (Chapter 5) (No. of Studies)			Included in Combination Therapies (Chapter 9) (No. of Studies)
			RCTs	CCTs	Non-Controlled Studies	
Qiang huo sheng shi tang 羌活胜湿汤	Yes	5	0	0	0	2
Shu feng huo xue tang 疏风活血汤	Yes	0	0	0	0	0
Juan bi tang 蠲痹汤	Yes	26	0	0	0	0
Tao hong si wu tang 桃红四物汤	Yes	0	0	0	0	1
Shen tong zhu yu tang 身痛逐瘀汤	Yes	0	1	0	0	1
Ban xia bai zhu tian ma tang 半夏白术天麻汤	Yes	0	0	0	0	0
Shen qi wan 肾气丸	Yes	0	0	0	0	0
Du huo ji sheng tang 独活寄生汤	Yes	0	0	0	0	0
Huang qi gui zhi wu wu tang 黄芪桂枝五物汤	Yes	0	0	0	3	0
Ba zhen tang 八珍汤	Yes	0	0	0	0	0
Fu ling wan 茯苓丸	No	45	0	0	0	0
Er chen tang 二陈汤	No	14	0	0	0	0
Dao tan tang 导痰汤	No	14	0	0	0	0
Kong xian dan 控涎丹	No	13	0	0	0	0
Wu ji san 五积散	No	11	0	0	0	0
Wu yao shun qi san 乌药顺气散	No	8	0	0	0	0
Shu jing tang 舒筋汤	No	6	0	0	0	0
Gun tan wan 滚痰丸	No	5	0	0	0	0
Ren shen san 人参散	No	4	0	0	0	0
Tong qi fang feng tang 通气防风汤	No	4	0	0	0	0
Gui zhi ji age gen tang 桂枝加葛根汤	No	0	1	0		2
Jing tong ke li 颈痛颗粒	No	0	1	0	1	8

Abbreviations: CCT, controlled clinical trial; RCT, randomised controlled trial.

literature and have also been evaluated in clinical studies. The lack of consistency indicates that during the long history of using CHM to treat CR-like conditions, there was some evolution in terms of the aetiology and pathogenesis of this condition from the Chinese medicine point of view, and that most of the CHM formulae evaluated in clinical studies did not use the names of classical formulae. Therefore, clinicians should refer to the commonly used herbs summarised in each category as a substitute.

Acupuncture-Related and Other Chinese Medicine Therapies

This section provides a summary of the evidence from Chapters 2, 3, 7, 8 and 9.

Acupuncture therapies have a long history of use for the clinical management of symptoms likely to be related to CR. Acupuncture, *tuina* 推拿 therapy and *daoyi* 导引 exercise have been included in all types of literature, with evidence showing these therapies are commonly used and effective in the management of CR. Electroacupuncture is recommended by clinical guidelines or textbooks and also supported by clinical research. There are other modern forms of acupuncture therapy, such as ear acupuncture, ear acupressure, abdominal acupuncture, etc., that have been evaluated by recent clinical research; however, more evidence is needed to confirm their treatment effects. Table 10.2 is a summary of these therapies from different types of evidence.

In order to summarise which acupuncture points were used for acupuncture treatment, the points that are recommended in Chapter 2 and used in the RCTs in Chapters 7 and 9 are presented in Table 10.3. The use of these points is cross-referenced to other clinical trial types and other chapters.

Most of the points recommended in Chapter 2 are also evidenced in both classical literature and clinical research, as shown in Table 10.3. The locations of these points are mainly in the cervical area and on the upper limbs.

Table 10.2. Summary of Acupuncture-Related and Other Chinese Medicine Therapies

Therapies	Included in Clinical Guidelines and Textbooks (Chapter 2)	Included in Classical Literature (Chapter 3) (No. of Citations)	Included in Clinical Studies (Chapters 7 or 8) (No. of Studies)			Included in Combination Therapies (Chapter 9) (No. of Studies)
			RCTs*	CCTs*	Non-Controlled Studies*	
Body acupuncture	Yes	295	10	0	10	30
Electroacupuncture	Yes	0	6	0	4	0
Heat-sensitive moxibustion	Yes	0	0	0	0	0
Ear acupressure	Yes	0	0	0	0	0
Cupping	Yes	0	0	0	0	4
Tuina 推拿 therapy	Yes	1	49	1	18	42
Daoyi 导引 exercise	Yes	8	0	0	2	8
Moxibustion	No	0	1	0	1	0
Warm needling	No	0	1	0	1	0
Ear acupuncture	No	0	2	0	0	0
Abdominal acupuncture	No	0	4	0	2	0

Abbreviations: CCT, controlled clinical trial; RCT, randomised controlled trial.

*Some studies used more than one intervention, e.g., acupuncture plus moxibustion. These are counted separately in this table.

Table 10.3. Summary of Acupuncture Points

Acupuncture Point	Clinical Guidelines and Textbooks (Chapter 2)	Classical Literature (Chapter 3) (No. of Citations)	Clinical Studies in Chapter 7 (No. of Studies)			Combination Therapies (Chapter 9) (No. of Studies)
			RCTs	CCTs	Non-Controlled Studies*	
EX-B2 *Jiaji* points 颈夹脊穴	Yes	0	11	0	8	2
Ashi points 阿是穴	Yes	0	5	0	6	10
GV14 *Dazhui* 大椎	Yes	2	10	0	4	14
BL10 *Tianzhu* 天柱	Yes	1	5	0	4	10
SI3 *Houxi* 后溪	Yes	13	4	0	0	13
BL11 *Dazhu* 大杼	Yes	0	4	0	1	1
SI11 *Tianzong* 天宗	Yes	15	1	0	3	13

(Continued)

Table 10.3. (*Continued*)

Acupuncture Point	Clinical Guidelines and Textbooks (Chapter 2)	Classical Literature (Chapter 3) (No. of Citations)	Clinical Studies in Chapter 7 (No. of Studies)			Combination Therapies (Chapter 9) (No. of Studies)
			RCTs	CCTs	Non-Controlled Studies*	
LI11 *Quchi* 曲池	Yes	57	2	0	2	19
LI4 *Hegu* 合谷	Yes	16	2	0	4	15
LI2 *Erjian* 二间	Yes	1	0	0	0	0
LI3 *Sanjian* 三间	Yes	1	0	0	0	0
LU5 *Chize* 尺泽	Yes	8	0	0	1	3
TE4 *Yangchi* 阳池	Yes	11	0	0	0	0
TE1 *Guanchong* 关冲	Yes	4	0	0	0	0
SI8 *Xiaohai* 小海	Yes	3	0	0	0	3
TE3 *Zhongzhu* 中渚	Yes	16	1	0	0	0
BL12 *Fengmen* 风门	Yes	1	0	0	0	0
GV16 *Fengfu* 风府	Yes	2	0	0	0	11
BL17 *Geshu* 膈俞	Yes	1	0	0	0	0
LR3 *Taichong* 太冲	Yes	7	0	0	0	0
GB21 *Jianjing* 肩井	No	40	2	0	2	24
LI15 *Jianyu* 肩髃	No	37	1	0	2	6
LI10 *Shousanli* 手三里	No	26	1	0	2	5
SI5 *Yanggu* 阳谷	No	20	0	0	0	1
SI2 *Qiangu* 前谷	No	16	0	0	0	0
SI4 *Wangu* 腕骨	No	15	0	0	0	0
TE5 *Waiguan* 外关	No	13	1	0	2	13
TE10 *Tianjing* 天井	No	13	0	0	0	1
LI12 *Zhouliao* 肘髎	No	11	0	0	0	1
TE2 *Yemen* 液门	No	10	0	0	0	0
TE14 *Jianliao* 肩髎	No	10	0	0	0	1

Abbreviations: CCT, controlled clinical trial; RCT, randomised controlled trial.

Limitations of the Evidence

Although we have made considerable effort to identify data from a wide range of sources, there may have been limitations from each of the data sources.

In Chapter 2, we synthesised current clinical guidelines and textbooks; however, these may not have comprehensively covered the information from some monographs. The analyses of the classical literature (Chapter 3) were based on the large sample of Chinese medicine books that are included in the *Zhong Hua Yi Dian* 中华医典 version 5. Our assessments indicated that this was the largest available digital resource at the time, but it did not include every Chinese medicine book published in the pre-modern era, so omissions were inevitable. The search processes employed a number of different search terms. Since CR was not considered a specific condition in history, we conducted a comprehensive search of not only known disease names but also combinations of terms that referred to the main symptoms of CR. However, we cannot be certain that all relevant citations were located and included in the analyses. Since the citations were written by multiple individuals throughout history, there have been changes in language usage and meaning, and errors may have crept into the processes involved in copying and printing manuscripts. Therefore, it is likely that the intended meanings of some citations have been misinterpreted and/or mistranslated. Similarly, the identities of some herbs may have changed over time and geographical location, so it is possible that regularisation errors have made in the allocation of scientific names. Moreover, it is not accurate to assume that the most frequently used herbs represent the most effective treatments, because there is no method of evaluating their efficacy. What they represent is a shortlist of herbs that could be considered for further research.

The clinical trial evidence was based on searches of multiple databases and resulted in thousands of search results. Since there was considerable variation in the conditions under which these trials were conducted, the age and disease severity of the participants, the frequency and duration of interventions, and the procedures used in data collection and analysis, it was not surprising that statistical heterogeneity tended to be "high" in some meta-analyses. Where possible, subgroup analyses were conducted, but they did not reduce the heterogeneity. The quality of the reporting of the methodological details of trial design and conduct was not adequate in many studies. Most of the included studies did not report proper random sequence generation. Among all the clinical studies, only one RCT applied participant blinding by using a placebo CHM as the comparator. All the other studies compared Chinese medicine therapies to conventional therapies, or compared a combination of Chinese medicine therapies and conventional therapies to conventional therapies alone, without a blinding approach. Due to the lack of blinding, the efficacy results achieved may not reflect the real therapeutic effects of Chinese medicine therapies. In addition, there was a lack of use of international guidelines" recommended outcome measures in most RCTs. The outcome measure of "effective rate" was the most common one; however, the criteria for judgement of "effectiveness" were not rigorous or consistent. As a result, except for the "effective rate", the sample sizes of the meta-analyses of other outcomes were insufficient, which also downgraded the certainty of evidence obtained from meta-analyses. It is worth highlighting that our evaluation identified one multi-centre, double-blinded RCT comparing oral CHM to a placebo. The design, sample size and outcome measures of this study fulfilled the requirements of clinical trial quality. Researchers should apply such designs in future trials to provide more rigorous clinical evidence.

For each category of evidence, frequency tables are provided that summarise the most commonly used interventions, including the herbal formula names, the herbal ingredients used in the formulae and the acupuncture points used in the clinical studies. Due to the large volume of available data, presentation of the details of every study was not feasible, and these tables only include the interventions that were the most frequently used. Lower frequency interventions may not be mentioned unless these featured prominently in the meta-analyses. Also, it should not be inferred that the most frequently used interventions were the most effective ones. The above limitations should be taken into consideration when interpreting the results included in the previous chapters.

Implications for Practice

Traditionally, the training of Chinese medicine practitioners largely relies on inheritance from the records in previous literature or senior practitioners" clinical experience. The evidence-based practice approach was not adopted in the development of most textbooks or clinical practice guidelines in Chinese medicine. In this research, we evaluated evidence from the classical literature and current clinical research, and provided information on how and to what extent treatments for CR were developed. The research provides evidence that supports the recommendations for the use of Chinese medicine therapies and identifies a gap between contemporary literature and current clinical practice in terms of some treatment methods.

According to all sorts of Chinese medicine literature, CR could be managed by oral CHM, topical CHM, acupuncture therapies, *tuina* 推拿 therapy, *daoyi* 导引 exercise or a combination of different types of Chinese medicine therapies. *Qi* stagnation and Blood stasis 气滞血瘀型 and wind-cold-dampness invasion 风寒湿型 are the most commonly seen Chinese medicine syndromes presented by patients who have CR. Prescribing CHM formulae and the selection of acupuncture points should take this syndrome differentiation into consideration. Relieving pain is one of the focuses of Chinese medicine therapies. Some toxic herbs are shown in the list of frequently used herbs in classical literature and modern clinical research, such as *fu zi* 附子/*wu tou* 乌头. Clinicians should pay attention to the toxicity of these herbs and comply with relevant regulations.

There is a lack of consistency in terms of CHM formulae across the different types of literature. Readers are advised to interpret the classical literature evidence with caution since the Chinese medicine aetiology of CR in history is different from the current understanding of this condition. It should be pointed out that some of the herbs recorded in classical literature may be restricted under the Convention on International Trade in Endangered Species of Wild Fauna and Flora (CITES), although they are not shown in the list of the most frequently used herbs (see Chapter 3). Readers who are looking for classical literature evidence are advised to comply with relevant regulations. On the other hand, there is consistent evidence on the use of acupuncture, *tuina* 推拿 therapy and *daoyi* 导引 exercise from all types of literature, although the quality of clinical studies limits the certainty of this evidence.

Implications for Research

Chinese medicine therapies are increasingly being evaluated through clinical trials, in line with the development of Western medicine. Our systematic analysis found that the Chinese medicine management of CR is encouraging, but high-quality evidence is lacking. Hence, there is a need for well-designed clinical trials of Chinese medicine interventions in order to provide accurate assessment of treatment effects. Furthermore, high-quality clinical trials are needed to address the following aspects.

General Trial Design

- RCTs should be designed with a rigorous methodology, with particular attention paid to adequate randomisation and allocation concealment;
- Since Chinese medicine therapies are commonly administered as add-on therapies to routine care/rehabilitation, efforts should be made to ensure the blinding of participants and practitioners with the use of placebos or sham controls;
- Considering that CR is a long-term condition, a follow-up phase is needed in order to evaluate the long-term effects of Chinese medicine therapies; and
- Clinical trial protocols should be registered in clinical trial registries or published prior to the start of RCTs to increase transparency in reporting.

Intervention and Control

- For CHM, authentication of raw materials should be described, and for manufactured products, reports should include the quantity of active constituents;
- Syndrome differentiation should be considered in study design to improve applicability in clinical practice; and
- Placebos or sham controls should be applied to ensure the blinding of participants and even practitioners.

Outcome Measures

Among all the clinical studies, the "effective rate" was the most commonly reported outcome measure. However, the criteria for judgement of "effectiveness" were not rigorous or consistent. Outcome measures recommended by international clinical guidelines are needed in order to accurately assess the efficacy of Chinese medicine therapies.

Reporting

- Research reports should follow the CONSORT statement with reference to the extension for herbal medicine[9] and STRICTA for clinical trials of acupuncture;[10]
- Individual modifications in the CHM formulae or acupuncture points used should be reported with more detail in order to instruct real-life clinical practice;
- Any modification or adjustment to the treatment method recommended by current clinical guidelines, and why and how these were done, should be addressed when reporting the results; and
- Adverse event information should be reported in more detail, and their causality and their relationship with the Chinese medicine therapy should be addressed.

Diversity was seen in the range of Chinese medicine therapies, both within and across the forms of evidence, reflecting the nature of Chinese medicine clinical practice. Future research should focus on the most promising findings identified and investigate the efficacy and safety of the therapies that are feasible to be widely used in clinical practice. Manual therapies (e.g., *tuina* 推拿 therapy and acupuncture) are more frequently used in the management of CR than CHM therapy. For manual therapies, more rigorous evidence is needed, although conducting double-blinded clinical trials to evaluate their efficacy and laboratory experiments to investigate their mechanisms is challenging.

References

1. Bono CM, Ghiselli G, Gilbert TJ, *et al.* (2011) An evidence-based clinical guideline for the diagnosis and treatment of cervical radiculopathy from degenerative disorders. *Spine J* **11**(1): 64–72.

2. Corey DL, Comeau D. (2014) Cervical radiculopathy. *Med Clin North Am* **98**(4): 791–799, xii.

3. Buxton S, Vermeersch J, Dartevelle S. Cervical radiculopathy. [cited 1 Oct 2019]. Available from: www.physio-pedia.com/Cervical_Radiculopathy#cite_note-Eubanks.2CJD-2.

4. Wang C, Tian F, Zhou Y, *et al.* (2016) The incidence of cervical spondylosis decreases with aging in the elderly, and increases with aging in the young and adult population: A hospital-based clinical analysis. *Clin Interv Aging* **11**: 47–53.

5. Woods BI, Hilibrand AS. (2015) Cervical radiculopathy: Epidemiology, etiology, diagnosis, and treatment. *J Spinal Disord Tech* **28**(5): e251–e259.

6. Abbed KM, Coumans JV. (2007) Cervical radiculopathy: Pathophysiology, presentation, and clinical evaluation. *Neurosurgery* **60**(1 Supp1): S28–S34.

7. Roth D, Mukai A, Thomas P, *et al.* (2009) Cervical radiculopathy. *Dis Mon* **55**(12): 737–756.

8. Kjaer P, Kongsted A, Hartvigsen J, *et al.* (2017) National clinical guidelines for non-surgical treatment of patients with recent onset neck pain or cervical radiculopathy. *Eur Spine J* **26**(9): 2242–2257.

9. Pandis N, Chung B, Scherer RW, *et al.* (2017) CONSORT 2010 statement: Extension checklist for reporting within person randomised trials. *BMJ* **357**: j2835.

10. MacPherson H, White A, Cummings M, *et al.* (2001) Standards for reporting interventions in controlled trials of acupuncture: The STRICTA recommendations. *Complement Ther Med* **9**(4): 246–249.

Glossary

Term	Abbreviation	Definition	Reference
95% confidence interval	95% CI	A measure of the uncertainty around the main finding of a statistical analysis. Estimates of unknown quantities, such as the odds ratio comparing an experimental intervention with a control, are usually presented as a point estimate and a 95% confidence interval. This means that if a study was repeated in other samples from the same population, 95% of the confidence intervals from those studies would contain the true value of the unknown quantity. Alternatives to 95%, such as 90% and 99% confidence intervals, are sometimes used. Wider intervals indicate lower precision; narrow intervals indicate greater precision.	http://handbook.cochrane.org
Acupuncture	—	The insertion of needles into humans or animals for remedial purposes.	WHO international standard terminologies of traditional medicine in the Western Pacific Region. World Health Organisation. 2007.

(Continued)

(*Continued*)

Term	Abbreviation	Definition	Reference
Allied and Complementary Medicine Database	AMED	Alternative medicine bibliographic database.	www.ebscohost.com/academic/ AMED-The-Allied-and-Complementary-Medicine-Database
Assessment Scale for Cervical Spondylosis	ASCS	An assessment scale that contains three sections to evaluate cervical spondylosis.	王晓红, 何成奇, 丁明甫, *et al.* (2005) 颈椎病治疗成绩评分表. *华西医学* (02): 232–233.
"Bone-setting" therapy	—	Known as 正骨疗法, this is a type of orthopaedic manipulation therapy used in traditional Chinese medicine.	—
China National Knowledge Infrastructure	CNKI	Chinese language bibliographic database.	www.cnki.net
Chinese Biomedical Literature database	CBM	Chinese language bibliographic database.	https://cbmwww.imicams.ac.cn
Chinese herbal medicine	CHM	Chinese herbal medicine.	—
Chinese herbal medicine iontophoresis	—	External application of Chinese herbal medicine using an iontophoresis apparatus.	—
Chinese medicine combination therapies	—	Two or more Chinese medicines from different therapy groups (Chinese herbal medicine, acupuncture therapies or other Chinese medicine therapies) administered together.	—
Chongqing VIP Information Company	CQVIP	Chinese language bibliographic database.	www.cqvip
Clinical Assessment Scale for Cervical Spondylosis	CASCS	An outcome measure assessing the symptoms, clinical signs and functional status of all types of cervical spondylosis patients.	张鸣生, 许伟成, 林仲民, 陈茵. (2003) 颈椎病临床评价量表的信度与效度研究. *中华物理医学与康复杂志* **25**(03): 25–28.

(*Continued*)

Term	Abbreviation	Definition	Reference
ClinicalTrials.gov	—	Clinical trial registry.	https://clinicaltrials.gov
Cochrane Central Register of Controlled Trials	CENTRAL	Bibliographic database that provides a highly concentrated source of reports of randomised controlled trials.	http://community.cochrane.org/ editorial-and-publishing-policy-resource/cochrane-central-register-controlled-trials-central
Convention on International Trade in Endangered Species of Wild Fauna and Flora	CITES	—	www.cites.org/eng/disc/text.php
Cumulative Index of Nursing and Allied Health Literature	CINAHL	Bibliographic database.	www.ebscohost.com/nursing/about
Daoyi 导引 exercise	—	*Daoyi* 导引 exercise refers to a series of body and mind unity exercises. It can be interpreted as a combination of gentle physical exercise and *qigong* therapy.	林定坤主编. (2016) 林定坤健体八段功. 广东教育出版社, 广州.
Effect size	—	A generic term for the estimate of the effect of treatment for a study.	http://handbook.cochrane.org
Excerpta Medica dataBASE	Embase	Bibliographic database.	www.elsevier.com/solutions/embase
Grading of Recommendations Assessment, Development, and Evaluation	GRADE	Approach to grading certainty (quality) of evidence and strength of recommendations.	www.gradeworkinggroup.org
Heterogeneity	—	(1) Used in a general sense to describe the variation in, or diversity of, participants, interventions and measurement of outcomes across a set of studies, or the variation in internal validity of those studies, and (2) Used specifically, as statistical	http://handbook.cochrane.org

(*Continued*)

(*Continued*)

Term	Abbreviation	Definition	Reference
		heterogeneity, to describe the degree of variation in the effect estimates from a set of studies. Also used to indicate the presence of variability among studies beyond the amount expected due solely to chance.	
I^2	—	A measure of study heterogeneity indicating the percentage of variance in a meta-analysis.	http://handbook.cochrane.org
McGill Pain Questionnaire	MPQ	A self-reporting measure of pain used for patients with a number of diagnoses.	Melzack R. (1975) The McGill Pain Questionnaire: Major properties and scoring methods. *Pain* **1**: 277–299.
Mean difference	MD	In meta-analysis: A method used to combine measures on continuous scales, where the mean, standard deviation and sample size in each group are known. The weight given to the difference in means from each study (e.g., how much influence each study has on the overall results of the meta-analysis) is determined by the precision of its estimate of effect; mathematically, this is equal to the inverse of the variance. This method assumes that all of the trials have measured the outcome on the same scale.	http://handbook.cochrane.org
Meta-analysis	—	The use of statistical techniques in a systematic review to integrate the results of included studies.	—

(*Continued*)

Term	Abbreviation	Definition	Reference
		Sometimes misused as a synonym for a systematic review, where the review includes a meta-analysis.	
Moxibustion	—	A therapeutic procedure involving ignited material (usually *moxa*) to apply heat to certain points or areas of the body surface for curing disease through regulation of the function of meridians/channels and visceral organs.	WHO international standard terminologies of traditional medicine in the Western Pacific Region. World Health Organization. 2007.
Non-controlled study	NCS	Observations made on individuals, usually receiving the same intervention, before and after an intervention, but with no control group.	http://handbook.cochrane.org
(Non-randomised) controlled clinical trial	CCT	An experimental study in which people are allocated to different interventions using methods that are not random.	http://handbook.cochrane.org
Northwick Park Neck Pain Questionnaire	NPQ	An outcome measure that measures neck pain and the consequent patient disabilities.	Vernon H, Mior S. (1994) The Northwick Park Neck Pain Questionnaire, devised to measure neck pain and disability. *Br J Rheumatol* **33**(12): 1203–1204.
Numeric Rating Scale	NRS	A subjective measure in which individuals rate their pain on an 11-point numerical scale. The scale ranges from 0 (no pain at all) to 10 (the worst imaginable pain).	Kjaer P, Kongsted A, Hartvigsen J, *et al.* (2017) National clinical guidelines for non-surgical treatment of patients with recent onset neck pain or cervical radiculopathy. *Eur Spine J* **26**(9): 2242–2257.
Other Chinese medicine therapies	—	Other Chinese medicine therapies including all traditional therapies except Chinese herbal	—

(*Continued*)

(*Continued*)

Term	Abbreviation	Definition	Reference
		medicine and acupuncture, such as *tuina* 推拿 therapy and *daoyin* 导引 exercise.	
Outcome Assessment System in the Treatment of Cervical Radiculopathy	OASTCR	An outcome measure developed by Zhu *et al.* that contains nine items with a total score of 35. 朱立国量表 (神经根型颈椎病疗效评定指标体系)	朱立国, 张清, 于杰, *et al.* (2009) 神经根型颈椎病疗效评定指标体系的效度分析. *中国中医骨伤科杂志* **17**(02): 22–23.
PubMed	PubMed	Bibliographic database.	www.ncbi.nlm.nih.gov/pubmed
Randomised controlled trial	RCT	A study in which a number of similar people are randomly assigned to two (or more) groups to test a specific drug, treatment or other intervention. One group (the experimental group) has the intervention being tested, the other (the comparison or control group) has an alternative intervention, a dummy intervention (placebo) or no intervention at all. The groups are followed up to see how effective the experimental intervention was. Outcomes are measured at specific times, and any difference in response between the groups is assessed statistically. This method is also used to reduce bias.	www.nice.org.uk/glossary
Risk of bias	—	Assessment of clinical trials to indicate whether the results may overestimate or underestimate the true effect because of bias in the study design or reporting.	http://handbook.cochrane.org

(*Continued*)

Term	Abbreviation	Definition	Reference
Risk ratio	RR	The ratio of risks in two groups. In intervention studies, it is the ratio of the risk in the intervention group to the risk in the control group. A risk ratio of 1 indicates no difference between comparison groups. For undesirable outcomes, a risk ratio that is less than 1 indicates the intervention was effective in reducing the risk of that outcome.	http://handbook.cochrane.org
Scoring System for Cervical Radiculopathy	SSCR	An outcome measure proposed by Tanaka *et al.* to evaluate pain, disability and neurological status. Known as 田中靖久颈椎病症状量表.	Tanaka Y, Kokubun S, Sato T. (1998) Mini-symposium: Cervical spine: (i) Cervical radiculopathy and its unsolved problems. *Curr Orthop* **12**(1): 1–6.
Short Form (36) Health Survey	SF-36	A 36-item patient-reported survey of patient health. The SF-36 is a measure of health status that is commonly used in health economics as a variable in the quality-adjusted life-year calculation to determine the cost-effectiveness of a health treatment.	Lins L, Carvalho FM. (2016) SF-36 total score as a single measure of health-related quality of life: Scoping review. *SAGE Open Med* **4**: 2050312116671725.
Summary of findings	SoF	Presentation of results and ratings of the quality of evidence based on the GRADE approach.	www.gradeworkinggroup.org
Teding Diancibo Pu lamp	TDP	A special electromagnetic spectrum lamp used in physiotherapy.	—
Tuina 推拿 therapy	—	Branch of traditional Chinese medicine concerned with the principles and clinical use of *tuina* (massage) therapy.	WHO international standard terminologies of traditional medicine in the Western Pacific Region. World Health Organization. 2007.

(*Continued*)

(*Continued*)

Term	Abbreviation	Definition	Reference
Visual Analogue Scale	VAS	A continuous measurement instrument for subjective characteristics or attitudes that cannot be directly measured, such as pain intensity.	Flynn D, Schaik VP, Wersch AV. (2004) A comparison of multi-item Likert and Visual Analogue Scales for the assessment of transactionally defined coping function. *Eur J Psychol Assess* **20**(1): 49–58.
Wanfang database	Wanfang	Chinese language bibliographic database.	www.wanfangdata.com
World Health Organization	WHO	WHO is the directing and coordinating authority for health within the United Nations system. It is responsible for providing leadership on global health matters, shaping the health research agenda, setting norms and standards, articulating evidence-based policy options, providing technical support to countries and monitoring and assessing health trends.	www.who.int/about/en
Zhong Hua Yi Dian 中华医典	ZHYD	The *Zhong Hua Yi Dian* "Encyclopaedia of Traditional Chinese Medicine" is a comprehensive series of electronic books on compact disk. It is the largest collection of Chinese electronic books and includes the major Chinese classical works, many of which are from rare manuscripts and are the only existing copies. These books cover the period from before the Tang dynasty to the period of the Republic of China (1911–1948).	Hu R, ed. (2014) *Zhong Hua Yi Dian* [*Encyclopaedia of Traditional Chinese Medicine*]. 5th edn. Hunan Electronic and Audio-visual Publishing House, Chengsha.

(*Continued*)

Term	Abbreviation	Definition	Reference
Zhong Yi Fang Ji Da Ci Dian 中医方剂大辞典	ZYFJDCD	Compendium of Chinese herbal formulae with over 96,592 entries derived from classical Chinese books. The Nanjing Chinese Medicine Institute compiled this and first published it in 1993.	Peng HR, ed. (1994) *Zhong Yi Fang Ji Da Ci Dian* [*Great Compendium of Chinese Medical Formulae*]. People's Medical Publishing House, Beijing.

Index

Evidence-based Clinical Chinese Medicine

(*Continued from page ii*)